# What I Didn't Expect

YSEULT D. LORSEILLE

# DEDICATION

To the eyes through which I have discovered the
path to my purpose.

To the one whose life changed the course of my
existence forever.

I love you, Isabelle.

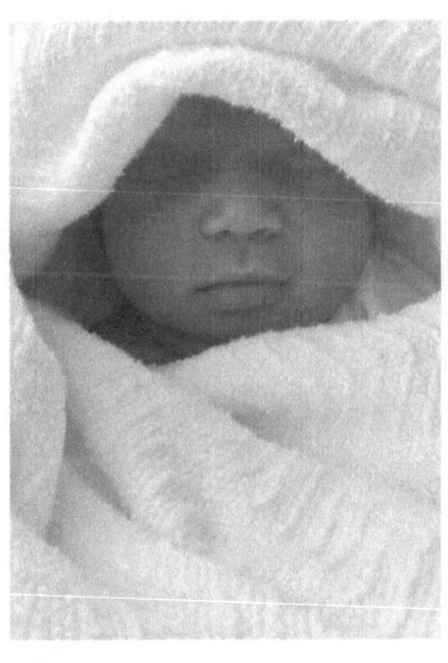

# ACKNOWLEDGMENTS


To the best P.A. I know, Dwayne A. Williams.
Thank you for your contributions to this book.  Your
medical wisdom and willingness to share your insight
have proven to be immeasurable and only come
second to your friendship.
Thank you, my friend.

# Table of Contents

# Prologue

Pregnancy was the most challenging experience of my life. After having my daughter, I wondered, was I the only one who sucked at pregnancy so much? Perhaps I did something wrong at some point in my life and now my pregnancy was God's way of punishing me. After all, isn't that the Christian belief behind the cause of labor pains? I was convinced I had to be the problem or in some way the reason behind this torture.

First of all, I never felt like I was glowing. I never felt like the women portrayed in those pregnancy commercials who rubbed their perfectly round bellies and smiled ear to ear from their anticipation of motherhood. Well, I guess that's not totally accurate. I was excited about having a baby and in the rare moments I was able to focus on anything other than pain or nausea, I felt love growing inside of me and I cherished every second of those rare occasions.

But, if we are to continue on the honesty train here, I couldn't wait for the process to be over. Every day, every month, every trimester brought along different difficulties that made my experience (again remember we're on the honesty train) simply horrible.

To those women who are experiencing difficulties throughout their pregnancy, my hope is that after you read my story you will never have to feel alone in your journey. Know that there are in fact many of us that have experienced the same or similar pregnancy issues. Some might even argue that an *easy* pregnancy isn't truly the norm and that most women do experience several bumps along the way. Stay strong ladies and be encouraged. Don't be ashamed to ask questions and never feel less adequate than the next woman who may appear to have it easier.

For those who have chosen to read simply seeking knowledge or perhaps to offer their support to their partner, family member or friend who may be experiencing a difficult pregnancy, I hope you will gain some understanding of the obstacles that many women face. Often in silence as we are taught that not feeling well is normal during pregnancy.

Here's to hoping at the very least, that speaking about my personal issues will empower more women to discuss their pregnancy struggles with their health care providers. So that one day, hopefully, they'll be more help for us.

Here are all the details of:
What I Didn't Expect

# WHAT I DIDN'T EXPECT

YSEULT D. LORSEILLE

<h1 style="text-align:center">1</h1>

# WHAT A PANG

3am one late night in November, I laid wide awake on my couch unable to fall asleep. I finally decided it was morning enough to get up and make breakfast. While rummaging through my kitchen I discovered that I didn't have the correct ingredients in my pantry to make the meal that I was suddenly craving. So, I got dressed and headed to the store to pick up some spaghetti noodles, pasta sauce and a pack of bacon. It didn't seem like an unusual breakfast option to me at all. What was clear was that meal seemed to be the only option to satisfy my sudden hunger and nothing was going to stop me from having my spaghetti with bacon.

I know, I know, I'd never heard of it before my brain conjured it up that morning either. But with food on the brain I was dressed and out the door within a matter of moments and headed to the 24-hour CVS which was conveniently located right across the street from my boyfriend's apartment. The perfect location to bring my ingredients and cook up an entire pot of pasta at 4am.

While at the pharmacy, I decided to pick up a pregnancy test, a double pack. My period was about 3 days late, so I figured I'd use a test this time and just save the other one for the next time my period was running a little late. Confused yet? Well, it was a trick I had played on myself for years. Whenever my period was late, I'd take a home pregnancy test and within hours of getting a negative result, my period would come! I have no idea why it happened that way, but it just did. So, there was no reason to think there would be any other outcome this time around.

But one pot of pasta and half a pack of bacon later, I was in for a shock. After tricking myself so many times, this time the joke was on me. I casually took the test and waited a minute or two for the result. But this time, that single line I was accustomed to seeing after peeping on the stick, was now accompanied by another line only a few seconds later. Now I'm the one who felt confused.

"It can't be… can it?" I asked myself. Well, it can, and I was pregnant! Several moments later, I figured I'd finally get out of the bathroom instead of standing there staring at the test results as if a message saying, 'Just Kidding!' was going to pop-up.

My disbelief that I was actually pregnant didn't allow the celebrating to begin yet. After all, I had done a great job up to that point at convincing myself that I couldn't get pregnant. I accepted the fact that motherhood might never be in my future. But there I was staring at now 2 tests (of course I had to take another one) and 4 perfectly clear blue lines.

Being in the bathroom for a ridiculously long time

now, my boyfriend came in. "Are you OK? I've been knocking on the door for the past 5 minutes." he said as his eyes scrolled down to the tests. I was holding them in one hand while I covered my mouth with the other.

"Yea, I'm fine." I replied while handing him the tests. I searched his face for a reaction as he took them from me. After looking at them for only a second, he immediately looked back up at me. "You're pregnant!" he said, excitedly.

OMG, he can see the lines too! Yay! For a moment I wasn't sure if my eyes were just going bad, but it was true. I was really pregnant!

"Yes! Yes, I am!" I replied. Finally, after wanting to be a mom for so long, it was going to happen. I ran out of the bathroom to call my mom and share the news.

***W.I.D.E Tip: Do something fun to commemorate the start of your pregnancy. You never know how the months will play out, so capturing the moment early on, before any of your symptoms kick in, may prove to be a good idea.***

A few days passed, and I began experiencing my first pregnancy symptom. The task of sleeping became nearly impossible; however, insomnia is not the symptom I'm referring to just yet. On the contrary, I was EXHAUSTED. I always felt like I could fall asleep anywhere at any moment during the day. But, falling asleep became impossible because I couldn't stop this feeling of extreme hunger. No, I don't mean a simple 'I'm hungry - let me grab a snack'. It was more like 'Dear God, why does it feel like I haven't eaten all week?!'

The hunger pains were so intense that they would keep me up at night. I tried to eat anything and everything I could to satisfy what I thought at the time was just hunger or possible pregnancy cravings. But no snack or 4 course meal would work and oddly enough, the pains only occurred at night. I would go to bed feeling exhausted then wake up a couple of hours later, starving.

I couldn't explain what I was feeling or why, so I just figured it was normal. After all, we've all seen or heard of pregnant women eating pickles with ice cream or snacking on almost anything all day. Maybe that's because they were as hungry as I was currently feeling. If that's the case, then I totally get it because there was nothing I wouldn't try eating to alleviate the pain.

Well, not so fast. You see, these weren't regular hunger pains or pregnancy cravings after all. These were more intense. **Hunger Pangs** as opposed to simply being hungry, occurs in your lower abdomen and is often only temporarily satisfied by food. The good thing was that the pains stuck around for about a week or so and finally, they subsided. Thank God because I desperately needed my sleep.

### *W.I.D.E Tip:  Staying hydrated may help to subside hunger pangs.*

Staying up half the night wasn't so bad at first. I found that there are a lot of good TV shows on during those hours that I would have not known about. I'd stay up watching cooking shows until about 4am, then I'd fall asleep only to wake up even more exhausted a couple of hours later. At this point I was nearing week

7 of pregnancy and was about to be introduced to another pregnancy symptom. One that would change the entire course of my pregnancy and pregnancy as I see it forever. Welcome, nausea.

## <u>HUNGER PANGS</u>

**<u>Definition:</u>** pain in the abdominal area due to increased contraction of an empty stomach or intestines.

- It is a very common condition during and prior to pregnancy.

**<u>Cause:</u>** may be due to hunger if it has been a long time since the last meal; however, it has many other causes including dehydration, eating the wrong foods, sleep deprivation & emotional state.

**<u>Symptoms:</u>** gnawing or rumbling in the stomach with abdominal pain coinciding with the contractions.

**<u>Diagnosis:</u>** usually a clinical diagnosis made by a physician after other causes of similar pain are not found to be the culprit.

**<u>Management:</u>** eating at regular intervals, choosing nutrient-dense food, increase sleep and hydration.

**<u>When To Call Your Doctor:</u>** severe pain, fever, dizziness and vomiting, as these symptoms may be indicative of another cause of abdominal pain.

**<u>Prognosis:</u>** they usually subside even without eating as the stomach gets to the level of emptiness.

# 2

# BUT, IT'S NOT MORNING?

My first sonogram was at 5 weeks and it didn't show much at the time. It only confirmed my pregnancy and I could see the newly formed sac that would host my baby for about 40 weeks. The next sonogram was scheduled for week 8 and what I saw on the monitor during that visit literally shocked me.

As I laid back on the examination table, the internal probe began searching my uterus. My doctor stopped moving the probe and turned the monitor to face me as he pointed at the screen. Right in front of my eyes I saw the tiniest outline of a human body. I could see the shape of a head, tiny little arms and a torso. The bottom half looked a bit mermaid-like, but even that was amazing. Its arms were flipping around like it wanted to swim.

I stared at the screen, then quickly down at my belly, then back up at the screen again and asked him "What is that?!"

"That's your baby", he said.

Duh, I thought. What kind of question was that? He must think I'm crazy. After all, that is why I was there in the first place. But it just seemed so incredible to me that just a few weeks ago at my first sonogram, I saw nothing. Now, I see a tiny, little, person. Alive and moving. It was remarkable. Although far too early for me to feel any of its movements, I couldn't wait for that first kick. The reality that at 33 years old I was finally going to be a

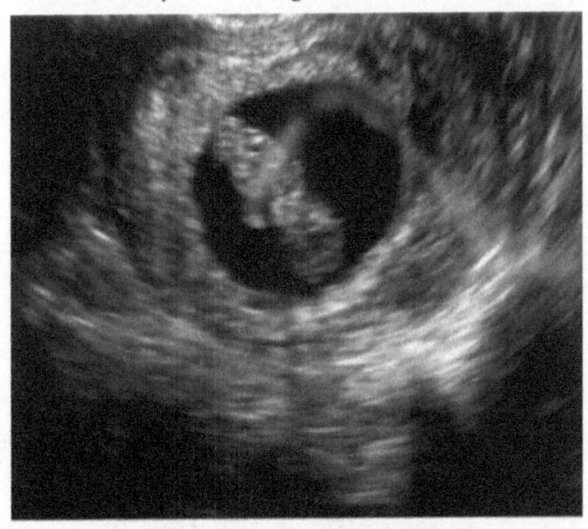

My baby's sonogram image at 8 weeks gestation. Just hanging out.

mom set in and so did the immediate and overwhelming feeling of unconditional love and protection. I was ready. I was… excited.

During that visit I mentioned to my doctor that I was starting to feel nauseous after taking my prenatal vitamins. Since the vitamins were vital to my and my baby's health, he encouraged me to continue taking them, but suggested that I try the gummy version instead. Those tend to be easier on the stomach. Also staying hydrated and taking the vitamins with food should help ease my nausea.

Here's where things start to get hairy. I'm not referring to body hair, although every hair follicle on my body seemed to have taken growth serum and I felt like a Chia Pet. I mean this is the part that forever altered my perception of pregnancy.

One morning while getting ready for work and taking a nice warm shower, I began to feel - queasy. Yea, queasy was a good word for it at the time. Nothing major. In fact, it didn't dawn on me yet that I was probably embarking on the next chapter of pregnancy that brought about **Morning Sickness**. So, casually I continued my morning routine and after showering I brushed my teeth. That's when I realized the thought alone of my toothbrush possibly touching the back of my throat sent my mind into a spiraling frenzy and I couldn't help but to just - vomit.

Ah, so this is morning sickness, I thought to myself. It wasn't so bad. Immediately after throwing up, I felt better and even a little hungry. I remember smiling and thinking to myself that finally, I would get to *feel* like I'm pregnant. What the hell was I thinking? Soon, I would be singing a very different tune.

In the days to follow my morning routine remained consistent. I'd wake up, shower, stare at my toothbrush for about 15 seconds hoping it would be nice to me today and not make me throw up, brush my teeth, throw up anyway, brush my teeth again, get dressed and off I'd go on my 1 and a half to 2-hour daily commute into New York City.

One morning while sitting on a crowded commuter train, my nausea started to creep back slowly. Confused, I thought this was strange because I had already completed my usual 'brush my teeth and throw up routine' that morning. So why was I nauseous again? Not thinking much of it, I closed my eyes and brushed it off as it being my acute sense of smell paired with riding a NYC train to be the culprit of my sudden nausea.

But a few minutes later, my eyes flew open again. It wasn't as simple as I could smell what everyone on the train had for breakfast that morning. Instead this was a full blown 'where's a bathroom because I'm going to need a sink ASAP' moment!

I quickly scrambled out of my seat saying excuse me at least a dozen times to my fellow passengers and made it to the bathroom just in time. Why am I throwing up again, I thought? My toothbrush was nowhere in sight this time. It was odd and to make it even stranger, within the few minutes it took me to get back to my seat, I was already nauseous again. I've got to get off this train, I thought. It had to be the reason why I was feeling like this.

That afternoon I ordered lunch even though my nausea **had** lingered for the better half of the day so far. I was hoping some soup would help to ease it a little. The receptionist called to tell me my food had arrived at **the front desk.**

I remember walking towards the reception area to collect my food, but quickly had to make a B line straight to the ladies' room instead. As I was throwing up, I remember thinking, Ok, I'm not brushing my teeth, I'm not on a crowded train, and it's not morning! Why the hell am I throwing up again for the 3rd time today? Rinsing my face off with some cold water, I quickly tried to gather myself as I walked out of the ladies' room. Still in my first trimester, I hadn't shared my news with any of my co-workers yet. So, I had to put on a smile, grab my food that's now been waiting for me at reception for an awkward 10 minutes and head back to my desk. All while realizing, my nausea was already creeping back. Again.

*W.I.D.E Tip: Be prepared to inherit someone else's nipples when you're pregnant. Your nipples may change in appearance so much, that they look like they should be on someone or maybe even something else.*
*I walked out of the shower one morning and was so shocked by what I saw in the mirror that I just stood there frozen. My nipples looked like they had tripled in size overnight and were now 10 shades darker. They looked like two bullseyes!*
*But don't worry ladies, after delivering (or breastfeeding) they'll return to their original appearance.*

## *MORNING SICKNESS*

**Definition:** nausea and/or vomiting usually lasting **up until 16 weeks gestational age (most common in the first trimester).**

**Pathophysiology:** increased sensitivity in the vomiting center of the brain to the increasing hormones of pregnancy (e.g., beta-hCG). The 4 chemicals in our brain that directly cause nausea and/or vomiting are serotonin, histamine, acetylcholine and dopamine. Therefore, some medications work by blocking these chemicals that trigger nausea and/or vomiting.

**Who's At Risk:** first time pregnancies, multiple gestations, migraine sufferers.

**When To Call Your Doctor:** if you develop weight loss, vomiting is excessive, you develop weakness or muscle cramps, the symptoms are worsening or persisting.

**Management:** All management options should be discussed with your primary care giver. Some options include but are not limited to:

• Lifestyle Modifications: **ginger**, high protein foods, small and frequent meals, avoiding trigger goods (e.g., spicy or fatty foods), increasing fluid intake. Women should keep a diary of triggers and foods that may provoke nausea and vomiting.

• **Pyridoxine (vitamin B6) with or without Doxylamine** is often **first-line medical management.**

• If no relief, antihistamines can be used (e.g., Dimenhydrinate, Meclizine or Diphenhydramine).

• 3rd line: dopamine-blocking agents (e.g., Metoclopramide or Promethazine). Ondansetron (serotonin blockers).

# 3

# I'M DIFFERENT

In the days and weeks to follow, my nausea and vomiting became more frequent. Day after day, I would dread getting out of bed because I knew what my day had in store for me. My nausea lingered even as I slept, so I would wake up restless, cranky, nauseous and just sad. By my 9th week I was vomiting at least 4-5 times a day. I didn't want to eat anything at all because everything made me nauseous. I had stopped taking my prenatal vitamins because they added to my nausea. Following my doctor's advice, I had tried switching to the gummy vitamins instead. He said they were supposed to be easier on the stomach. Nope, not on my stomach. Everything made me sick. Food, water, air, you name it. If my body ingested it in any way, it would eventually make me vomit.

At that point I began feeling very weak. My constant nausea wasn't allowing me to eat and properly supply the nutrition that my baby and I needed. The very little that I was able to eat would never stay down.

Can you imagine that feeling? It was horrible. Prior to getting pregnant, I was such a foodie. I loved eating and trying new foods. When I found out I was pregnant, I couldn't wait to have a good reason to stuff my face with tons of delicious varieties of food. I would have had a great excuse for it too, I thought. But sadly, that wasn't my reality at all.

Most women are worried about gaining too much weight during pregnancy, while my concern was not gaining enough. Not being able to properly supply my body with the nutrients it needed to keep my baby growing and safe made me feel, incapable. Why am I so different I kept asking myself? I'd never heard of other women complaining of the extreme nausea I was feeling. They always made morning sickness sound 'cute'. But there was nothing cute about the way I was feeling.

I tried everything I could or was suggested to me to combat the nausea and vomiting. From drinking ginger ale to eating ginger cookies, ginger candy, raw ginger, seltzer water, bland foods, soups, crackers, the list went on and on. I literally tried everything I could, but *nothing* helped.

My biggest enemy seemed to be water. I couldn't believe it. How can water make me feel so sick? The thought alone of drinking it would make me nauseous immediately. Before pregnancy, I loved drinking water. I was never a big fan of sodas or most juices. Water was my thing, but now, it appeared my love affair with it was totally over.

Oh, but wait, there's a catch. You see, while I couldn't stomach drinking any water, it was also a key component of what my body needed to help ensure a healthy pregnancy. Both my doctor and my boyfriend would tell me to make sure I drank at least a gallon of water a day. Ha, yeah right! I could barely get beyond a sip a day.

Do you know what happens when someone is not drinking enough water? You of course become dehydrated which under normal circumstances is never a good thing. But it's even worse and more dangerous when you're pregnant.

By week 12, I was checking the pregnancy app I had downloaded onto my phone constantly to see when I could anticipate feeling better and my morning sickness would finally go away. According to the app, some women would start to feel better at this point in their pregnancy. By the second trimester (which again per my app was allegedly going to be the best one), the queasiness is supposed to completely subside. So why was I still feeling so miserable? Did I get my dates/weeks wrong? Maybe I'm not actually 12 weeks yet, I figured. I knew something I did wrong had to be the reason why I was still feeling so sick. Why else would my experience so far be so different than what I was expecting?

***W.I.D.E Tip: Many women I know suffer from severe heartburn during pregnancy. My battle with heartburn only lasted a week or so and I was able to get relief by using over the counter heartburn medication. Ranitidine tablets 150 mg did the trick for me. If you're suffering with heartburn, ask your doctor if it might work for you.***

# 4

# IS THIS SAFE?

One of my co-workers was pregnant at the same time that I was. She was a month ahead of me and had already announced to everyone at the office that she was expecting. I remember thinking to myself, how does she do it? She didn't look sick at all. Actually, she was kind of glowing. I decided to share my then pregnancy secret with her, hoping that she would share her secret with me as to how she was making it look so easy.

I personally felt like I could no longer hide why I was getting up from my desk to run to the ladies room almost every hour. During our quick talk, she shared with me that although she had some queasiness in her first trimester, she never actually threw up. Her nausea was gone after a few weeks and she felt completely fine afterwards. I smiled and pretended like I wasn't already way beyond that point of my pregnancy and yet I was still sick as a dog.

She also shared that she had a friend who was very

sick during the early stages of her pregnancy and that her doctor prescribed her something that alleviated her nausea. Those words were like music to my ears. I told myself if my nausea persisted, I would call my doctor to ask him for help.

At 13 weeks I'd decided to put my foot down, stop suffering in silence and demand help to fight this constant nausea and vomiting. Up to that point, every time I'd complain about symptoms to my doctor, he would just try to assure me that I was experiencing a normal pregnancy symptom and that like most women who have been in his care many times before, it would soon pass. Well, I was tired of throwing up a dozen times a day, feeling weak, not wanting to get out of bed and just miserable. I vomited so frequently that most of the time, the only thing coming up was bile.

I called my doctor and reluctantly, he prescribed me Ondansetron. An anti-nausea medication usually prescribed to cancer patients after receiving chemotherapy. The medication was safe to use during pregnancy and had been found to be helpful in some cases of extreme morning sickness. Eager to get my prescription filled, I left my office and headed straight to the pharmacy.

After picking up my prescription, I headed home eager to take the first dose with the hopes it would soon make me feel better. I decided to do some research on the drug on my commute home. The reviews were mixed. Wondering if this was going to be safe for my baby, I decided to call my Uncle, a doctor that specialized in general medicine. Speaking with him eased my concerns. He explained that not only was the medication safe to use during pregnancy, but that it was often prescribed to women to help alleviate their nausea. He made me feel less guilty about needing help and in that moment, I didn't feel so alone.

The week to follow was probably the best week out of my entire pregnancy. Only taking my prescription when needed, my nausea had passed, and I was finally able to keep some food down! I woke up in the morning feeling great and had the energy now to make myself look presentable. Prior to that, I barely had enough strength to get myself ready for work. Caring about what I wore and how I looked was the least of my problems. But for now, I was feeling great. Finally, I thought, finally I can enjoy this.

That feeling was short lived. The following week, I took my prescription as usual in the morning. But one morning after taking it, I quickly realized my nausea didn't go away. In fact, it became more intense as the day progressed and eventually, you know what happened next, I threw up. Ugh! Why?! Why am I throwing up again?

Frustrated, I stopped taking the medication after the second pill that day failed to get rid of my nausea. Out of the 30 pills I was prescribed, I had only taken a total of 9. To me it didn't make sense to continue taking them. Why would I continue putting this drug in my body if it wasn't even working anymore?

I felt so depressed and so defeated. Just a week ago I was starting to feel better and thought I was finally going to enjoy my pregnancy. But now I was back to the constant nausea and vomiting that plagued me before. I felt heartbroken and confused. I was convinced the Ondansetron was going to work. It worked for other women and made them feel better, so why did it stop working for me? I was so angry that all I wanted to do was cry. But there was no time for tears.  I was at work and had things to do. Work didn't stop because I wasn't feeling well, and no one was going to understand or feel sorry for a pregnant woman who was crying over feeling sick anyway.

# 5

# GETTING ON MY NERVES

Around 16 weeks nausea and vomiting went on a short hiatus, but there was another pregnancy ailment that was about to make its grand entrance. One day I was doing some house work, when out of nowhere I felt the sharpest, most electrifying pain that I had ever felt in my female parts. I mean it felt like I was in the middle of a thunderstorm and a bolt of lightning hit me in the vagina. The pain stopped me dead in my tracks and I let out a yell like Drew Barrymore did in the opening scene of Scream.

"Ouch" I screeched while dropping the broom and grabbing my crotch. It was like my baby had suddenly decided to take up guitar playing, and my urethra was the closest string that she could use for practice.

I called my doctor and he told me what I was feeling was normal and that I was probably experiencing **Round Ligament Pain**.

"It's normal. It will pass." he said. Well several days and long agonizing nights later, the pain was still coming on quite often. It always seemed to catch me by surprise at the most inconvenient places. Imagine spending 3 - 4 hours commuting plus another 8 and a half hours with your colleagues every day, when at any moment your growing baby could kick you in the vagina stopping you dead in your tracks and causing you to scream like a lunatic while grabbing your crotch. It made for a very interesting work day!

I had tried everything to alleviate the pain. I remember hanging upside down on my couch with my legs up to God for hours hoping that position would take away the pressure I was feeling in my pelvis.

At one point I thought maybe I had a UTI (even though my tests were negative) and that I should drink as much cranberry juice as I could stomach - because by now my nausea and vomiting were already back from vacation, fully rested and ready to give me hell again. But nothing worked.

I researched online daily hoping to find an answer as to what this crazy pain was all about. My sonogram technician once suggested that perhaps I had scar tissue from my prior abdominal surgery and now, as my uterus grew, it could be causing the pain. She suggested I try a belly band. I bought 2 different kinds, and neither were able to do the trick as the pain persisted. I could barely walk without slouching over from the constant discomfort.

Much later down the road, as in way after my pregnancy, I had finally found my answer. What I was experiencing was **Pudendal Nerve Pain (PNP)**. It's an acute pain that once you experience it, you never forget it and you pray that you don't randomly feel it again. Especially not somewhere as inconvenient as being on a crowded train during your morning rush hour commute like I did. I'm pretty sure I got a lot of stares when I let out a squeal and grabbed my crotch that morning. But then again, maybe they just thought I was giving my best Michael Jackson impersonation? Who knows, but I can tell you at that moment I couldn't care less. All I felt was that pain and I needed to place my hand down there to prevent my baby from kicking her way out.

I wish I could say that eventually the pain went away, but it never really did. As the months went by, they became more sporadic, but I felt PNP well into my third trimester. Eventually, my co-workers just got used to me randomly grabbing my crotch. I'm just thankful no one called HR!

## *ROUND LIGAMENT PAIN*

**Definition:**   pain at the location of the round ligament.

• A very common condition experienced during the second trimester of pregnancy.

**Cause:**   the round ligament is a thick ligament that surrounds and supports the uterus (womb) as it grows during pregnancy. Stretching of the ligament as the uterus grows can cause pain due to spasm of the round ligament or irritation of the nerve fibers surrounding it.

**Symptoms:**   sharp or jabbing pain or sensations that most commonly occur on the right side of the abdomen, groin or pelvis and lasts for a few seconds. It most commonly occurs with sudden movements that causes the ligament to tighten abruptly, such as rolling over in bed, sneezing, coughing, upon waking or with strenuous activity.

**Diagnosis:**   it is usually a clinical diagnosis made

by your physician after other causes of similar pain are not found to be the culprit.

**Management:** changes in position or avoiding sudden movements when possible may alleviate the pain. Exercises to strengthen the core muscles may reduce the pain. Consult with your doctor on which exercises are safe. If you have to sneeze or cough, bending and flexing your hips before coughing or sneezing may help. With the consultation of your physician, acetaminophen may be used for moderate to severe pain.

**When To Call Your Doctor:** pain lasting a few minutes, severe pain, fever or chills, difficulty walking or burning with urination as these symptoms may indicate other problems, such as an infection.

**Prognosis:** the pain is usually mild and self-limited as your body adjusts to the changes during pregnancy.

## *PUDENDAL NEURALGIA (NERVE PAIN)*

**Definition:** pain along the distribution of the pudendal nerve. The pudendal nerve runs between the anus to the genitals.

• It is a very common condition that is most commonly experienced during the second trimester of pregnancy.

**Cause:** entrapment, pinching, compression or irritation of the pudendal nerve.

**Symptoms:** pain (aching, stabbing, sharp or burning) along the distribution of the pudendal nerve - vulva, vagina, clitoris, perineum (the space between the anus and the vulva) and rectum. This pain is often described as lightning with sudden onset that can be unpredictable. The pain can be worsened with sitting.

This pain can sometimes be so extreme that it can be difficult to complete everyday tasks. It may sometimes cause pain with bowel movements or with urination.

**Management:**  physical    therapy    and acetaminophen, as needed.

*W.I.D.E Tip:  it's probably not a good idea to find out the sex of your baby while you're driving. The nurse called with the results from our Noninvasive Prenatal Testing (a blood test used to determine the likeliness of certain genetic disorders and provides the baby's gender). My boyfriend nearly crashed his car when she said, "It's a girl!" Hahaha, poor guy. Little did he know that our daughter would soon have him wrapped around her little finger.*

# 6

## *IT* WON'T BE VIABLE

Although it felt like most of the time I was in pain or having some sort of discomfort; one of the things I truly enjoyed during my pregnancy were my routine doctor's visits. My boyfriend and I always looked forward to seeing and hearing our daughter's strong heartbeat. We would watch her roll around and sometimes even catch her sucking on her thumb. I wish I could pause those moments and make them last forever. When I saw her inside of me, I would forget about everything and things would make sense again.

I had a wonderful group of medical professionals taking care of me and my baby. They always greeted me warmly and made me feel special. Even though I'm sure I was one out of a dozen women they probably examined that day, they never made me feel that way. Especially the nurses. God bless nurses. They always comforted me, answered my questions and always made sure that I got to leave with a new sonogram picture after every visit. I don't think I would have made it beyond my second trimester had it not been for the great team of professionals I had in my corner.

One day afterwork, I headed down to Brooklyn to get my hair done. On my short walk from the train station to the hair salon, I stopped to pick up a snack to eat when I got there. I had been feeling OK for a few days and was glad that I could finally pamper myself a little. Lord knows I needed it. I looked a hot mess. I had to schedule everything around how I felt. No plans were ever promised as I never knew how I'd feel on the day of.

I arrived at my hair salon and ate my snack as I waited my turn. I chatted with my hairstylist and caught her up on all things regarding my pregnancy since I hadn't seen her in so long. Normally, I'd have a hair appointment at least every 2 weeks. But on that day, I hadn't been there in almost 4 months!

Halfway through getting my hair done I felt a strange feeling come over me. A sudden heat flash shot up from my feet all the way up my body and as soon as it reached my head, I instantly became dizzy. It came on so suddenly that my immediate reaction was to quickly jump up from the styling chair and cradle my belly. Almost like I was using my arms to protect my baby from an unseen predator.

"Are you OK?" my hairstylist asked. I could hear the panic in her voice as she reached her hand out to help me from falling over. I took several deep breaths trying to calm the feeling away. "I think so", I replied as I sat back down still feeling the room spinning around me.

Everyone at the salon quickly tended to me making sure I was alright. I was embarrassed that I was causing a scene and just wanted to get back to getting my hair done. They gave me water and placed a cool rag on my forehead, but nothing seemed to help.

Suddenly, an intense feeling of nausea overcame me. I didn't even have enough time to make it to the restroom. A woman at the salon saw the expression on my face and knew what was about to happen. Quickly, she grabbed a plastic bag and handed it to me. Seconds later, I threw up while still sitting in the styling chair. But that was not going to be the end of it.

I then began to feel a pain in my stomach that I'd never felt before. It was a sharp, stabbing pain that seemed to come on in waves. I cried out in pain hunched over while holding onto my stomach. I remember hearing a woman's voice in the background yell out "She's in labor, call the ambulance!"

"No", I whispered unable to speak up from the pain. "Please God, no. It can't be." I was only 5 months pregnant I thought, as a sudden sense of fear rushed through my body and the tears began falling, before I could catch them.

Now completely hunched over, I got my bearings together for a moment and asked that instead of calling for an ambulance, that someone please take my cellphone and call a family member to come and escort me to a nearby hospital instead. I didn't want to leave in an ambulance alone. The hair salon was in the neighborhood where I grew up in Brooklyn, so having a family member who still lived nearby come and escort me to the ER just made sense. Not only for support but also as my advocate.

My boyfriend was at work over 2 hours away from my location and I knew I needed to get to the hospital immediately. It would have taken too long for him to get to me. The ladies at the salon called my brother.

Moments later, he had arrived and we were headed to the nearest emergency room.

Upon arrival, the ER staff quickly took me into a room. The pain had become so intense that I could barely focus to make out what anyone was saying to me. It felt as though I was drifting in and out of consciousness. Every time I opened my eyes, through a squint I could see a new family member had arrived to support me. Thank God. I was terrified and felt some relief knowing I wasn't alone.

Several tests later, the ER doctor suggested that I be transported to my hospital where I had planned to give birth. This way I may be seen by my own doctor. He didn't elaborate much on what he thought was causing my pain but made it clear that I would need to be further evaluated.

It felt like I was in a bad dream. Everything was a blur. I remember that night only in flashes. A flash of being strapped into the back of an ambulance with one brother by my side. A flash of my boyfriend's face staring through the back of the ambulance window as the doors closed and he was getting in his car to follow us. A flash of my other brother walking next to my stretcher as we arrived at the next hospital.

I can also remember the nurses. Not their faces, but their voices. Calm, soothing voices. They asked me questions, hooked me up to an IV, took my and my baby's vitals, strapped some sort of monitor around my belly and assured me I was going to be OK.

Several hours later and still unable to provide me with any reason for the pain I was in, the doctor started me on a dose of Morphine. What was clear was that they needed to manage the pain and get me comfortable asap.

As the medicine flowed through the IV and into my body, the tears started to fall again. I remember thinking to myself, this can't be good for my baby. What's wrong with me? What's wrong with my body? As I drifted off to sleep, I remember hearing the screams coming from a woman in labor in the room next door. That's when it hit me, I was in the Labor and Delivery unit of my hospital, at only 20 weeks.

I was admitted into the hospital for 5 days during that visit. Mostly to get fluids as I was extremely dehydrated. In addition to the fluids, I was being kept comfortable with Morphine and intravenous anti-nausea medication until the doctors could determine the reason behind my severe discomfort. Even on medication the vomiting continued while I was in the hospital. I became increasingly sad and I could feel a state of depression starting to take over my body. It was so hard to explain what I was feeling when the doctors themselves couldn't find a reasonable explanation for my pain.

There were several tests ordered. Among them was a urinalysis. The results showed I had traces of blood in my urine which could be a sign of **Kidney Stones**. Just what I needed, I thought to myself. As if this pregnancy couldn't get any worse, now I'm going to have to pass a stone too? I always heard that passing a kidney stone was like labor pains. Now it looks like I'll get to experience both! Ugh, why me? The thought of it made me nervous but having a stone would be a good explanation for the pain and why it felt like my baby was kicking me in the kidney.

The doctor ordered an ultrasound. I tried to lay flat while the technician performed the examination, but I couldn't help but to squirm around and jump from the quick sudden jolts of pain on the right side of my body.

"I'm sorry" I said to the technician. "It just that it feels like she's kicking me in my kidney."

We both laughed but I was serious. The technician decided to roll the probe around to the area I was pointing to and she was shocked! "Oh, my goodness, she is kicking you in the kidney!" she said in disbelief. "I told you.", I replied trying to laugh through the pain.

I looked over at the monitor and I could see my little girl going to town on my organs. I can't lie it made me laugh. It was so cute to see that tiny little foot jabbing at my insides with no regard to the pain she's putting her mommy in. The technician couldn't print images from her machine, but I had my cell phone and was able to snap a picture. I smiled and for a moment, I felt better.

Fortunately, the sonogram revealed no signs of a kidney stone. The bad part was that now we were back to square one. After 5 days in the

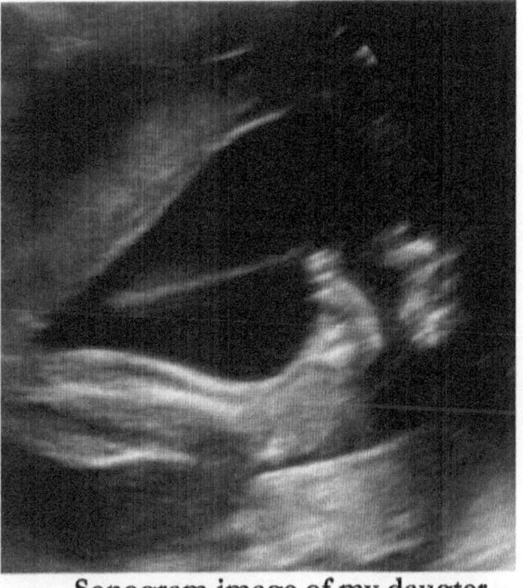

**Sonogram image of my daugter kicking away at my right kidney.**

hospital, the doctors decided to send me home. Que my waterworks. Of course I started crying again. There I was still with no answers and I was being sent home with a prescription for Oxycodone. God, I thought. How messed up can my body be that I'm being prescribed such a strong pain medication while pregnant? Surely the doctors knew the risks behind the medication, but I guess having me take it was less risky than the harm I'm already causing on my body from being in this much pain. I had a gut feeling things were only going to get worse after I was discharged, and I was right.

Still in pain, I left the hospital and made my way down to my family's house. My mother and brother accompanied me on the trip while my boyfriend went back to work. It felt like the pain had gotten worse the moment I sat in the car. I then realized, the Morphine that had been keeping me somewhat comfortable over the past several days was beginning to wearing off.

By the time we arrived at the house, it was as though time had rewinded itself and I was right back at the hair salon feeling the same intense, stomach cradling pain I was in 5 days ago. My brother ran out to quickly fill my prescription hoping it would provide me some relief. I took the first dose but it didn't alleviate the pain at all. We were't even home a full hour yet and my mother had to call for another ambulance.

I was once again going in and out of consciousness from the pain and could barely speak. The next thing I remember was being strapped in the back of an ambulance heading to yet another emergency room. It was like reliving a scary dream that I couldn't wake myself up from.

Once there, I was placed on a stretcher and now a third set of nurses and doctors began running tests on me. This hospital experience was very different from the others. I can remember being injected in the arm with a huge needle to administer Morphine. The shot itself was so painful but I didn't care. I just needed the pain to go away. This time however, it didn't work.

A few agonizing hours later, they gave me another shot in the arm and that one didn't work either. Now remember how I spoke about the nurses who took care of me before? How comfortable they made me feel and how although I may not be able to remember their faces, I can distinctly remember their voices? Well, not this time. This time there were 2 nurses that I remember clearly and for 2 very different reasons.

The first nurse casually told me that I was in fact having contractions. When she said it, my eyes which were closed from the pain flew open and my head turned in the direction she was standing and I stared her directly in her eyes.

"What did you just say?" I asked needing to make sure I heard her correctly.

"You're having contractions" she repeated, very matter of factly.

Shocked by her words, I asked her what that meant for me, and for my baby. Her reply gave me chills. Without a single crack in her voice she said "Should there become a need to deliver your baby at this time, *it* would not be viable."

I wish I could put into words how I felt at that moment. But nothing written in black and white would do my feelings any justice. I fell into a daze helplessly staring into space. The room seemed to have gotten very quiet even though everyone was still there. The nurse, my brother, even the machines were still beeping, but it's like everything became silent and all I could hear was the sound of my own heartbeat.

Almost as though God could read my mind and knew I needed a lifeline to save me from my own thoughts, he sent me an angel to pull me out of the darkness I was quickly sinking into. I heard a voice call my name. It was another nurse. She had overheard what the first nurse had just told me while walking into the room. I'm assuming the blank look on my face made her come over to me.

She looked at me lying helplessly on the stretcher dazed and in pain and calmly whispered "You should leave this hospital. You won't get the proper care for you and your baby here. Go where they'll be able to take better care of you."

Completely surprised by her words I also suddenly felt encouraged. I was not about to just lay there and let my baby die. I knew what I had to do. While sitting myself up, I turned to her and said "Thank you. You don't have to tell me twice."

I disconnected the monitor I had strapped around my stomach, fought to stand on my feet and asked that I be released, immediately. Moments later, my brother and I were once again headed back to my delivery hospital which I had just been discharged from only hours ago.

About an hour after arriving and getting setup with my 3$^{rd}$ IV line in 24 hours, the attending physician came in to have a brief conversation with me. He decided to try a different approach to determine the cause of my pain. With my approval, he suggested we try performing an abdominal CT Scan so they can really see what's going on inside of me. Under normal circumstances, CT Scans are not usually performed on pregnant women due to the risk factors of exposing the growing fetus to the radiation. But in my case, it was all about the risk to benefit ratio. The doctor explained that it would be my choice whether or not they would perform the exam.

After asking lots of questions, including what amount of radiation my baby would be exposed to and having him fully explain the chances of any complications, I decided to go ahead with the scan. I understood the stress my body was experiencing from the pain was becoming more dangerous for my baby by the minute. You hear it all the time that stress is not good for your body. Well it's out right dangerous when you're pregnant. Getting the CT scan felt like the right thing to do in order to get answers. I wanted to feel better. Not only for myself but for my baby. Maybe then I could start enjoying my remaining months of pregnancy.

Well, guess what the results from the scan showed? That I was extremely constipated. I mean I was literally full it! Stop laughing. Yes, I know it's gross but hey, what else do you expect from a 5 month pregnant woman who can't hold down any water? Being unable to drink water meant dehydration. Dehydration then leads to constipation. All of my pregnancy ailments were perfectly aligned to give me a well rounded miserable pregnancy. Yay, me!

While still uncertain if the constipation was the cause behind my pain, the doctors started me on lots more intravenous fluids, laxatives and anti-heartburn medication. Within a day, the contractions had stopped and I was finally beginning to feel better. This time I was discharged with a prescription for Oxycodone/Acetaminophen. Luckily, I never had to take one. I couldn't stop thinking about the amount of medications my baby had already been exposed to. I didn't want to unnecessarily expose her to anymore. If the pain was **bearable**, I'd just suck it up.

## ***KIDNEY STONES***

**Definition:**    hard deposits of minerals and salts in the urinary tract.

• Stones in the ureters (the tube that carries urine from the kidney to the bladder for storage) are twice as likely to occur in pregnant patients.

• Approximately 85-90% of pregnant patients with kidney stones develop symptoms in the second or third trimester of pregnancy because spontaneous passage of stones is more difficult at these stages of pregnancy.

• Kidney stones are one of the most common causes of non-pregnancy related abdominal pain in pregnant women that requires being admitted to the hospital.

**Cause:**    dehydration is the most important risk factor for the development of kidney stones.

**Symptoms:**    renal colic – sudden, constant upper lateral back or flank pain that may radiating to the groin or anteriorly to the labia. This pain may make it difficult to find a comfortable position. Other symptoms include nausea, vomiting as well as increased urinary frequency, urgency or blood in the urine.

• Pain varies with location of the stone (e.g., flank, mid abdominal pain or groin). It is not usually associated with fever.

**Management:**    once diagnosed by your health care provider, options include symptomatic management, such as increased fluid intake and pain medications (as determined by your medical provider). If stones are large, then additional options are discussed with the patient.

**Prevention:** increased fluid intake during pregnancy is the best prevention for all forms of kidney stones.

**When To Call Your Doctor:** if you develop fever, severe nausea or vomiting, persistent or severe abdominal pain, cramps, burning with urination or chills as it may indicate an infection or another abdominal process.


## *URINARY TRACT INFECTION (UTI)*

**Definition:** infection along the lower urinary tract (urethra and the bladder).

**Pathophysiology:** usually an ascending infection of the lower urinary tract from the urethra. Bacteria are the most common cause of UTI. The anatomical changes in pregnancy put women at increased risk for UTI development.

**Clinical Manifestations:** irritative symptoms – dysuria (burning) as well as increased urinary frequency, & urgency (sudden extreme urge to urinate). Blood in the urine & tenderness above the pubic bone may occur.

• Antibiotics that are safe in pregnancy (as discussed with your medical provider).

• Many home remedies are tried but increased fluid intake and frequent voiding are the most proven ways to reduce the incidence of UTIs.

**When To Call Your Doctor:** if you develop flank pain, fever, chills, abdominal cramps, nausea, vomiting or back pain as this may indicate the infection in the upper urinary tract or some other process.

# 7

# I DESERVE A BREAK

As the weeks went by, I felt better. Not great, but better. My nausea and vomiting still lingered a bit but I wasn't throwing up as often. Maybe once or twice a week. That was nothing compared to what I was experiencing before, so I wasn't complaining. I was just starting my third trimester and I started shopping for baby clothes, thinking of names for my baby girl and trying to enjoy my pregnancy a little. My emotions were all over the place but hey, at least I wasn't in pain. It still felt like she was tap dancing on my urethra from time to time. That seemed to be her thing and she never gave it up my whole pregnancy.

Nearing month 7, my boyfriend and I went to my next doctor's appointment. I was so excited as we were planning to travel in a few days to visit family and I was hoping my doctor would give me the greenlight to fly. I desperately needed a break and I thought a short trip would do the trick. I could take a break from my agonizing daily commute which seemed to be getting harder and harder by the day. Hopefully, I'd also be able to get some sleep.

My nights were starting to become restless again. Mostly caused by insomnia, but also my little girl was taking up a lot more room. She was a night owl with her prime-time party hours being 12am to 4am. That meant mommy would have to stay up too. She would move around so much that I eventually just got up and started doing housework. I might as well make good use of the time awake.

Seeing that I was feeling better, my doctor gave me the OK to travel. Thank goodness, because we had already booked our tickets and I had planned on giving my best devastated pregnant woman performance in his office, complete with tears, sobbing and rolling around on the floor if he said I couldn't go.

A few days later we were off to Salt Lake City. We booked a connecting flight which included a short layover in Denver. Normally, I would never book a connecting flight unless there were no other options. But something told me breaking up the over 5-hour direct flight would be a good idea for me and I was right.

We had an early morning flight, so we stopped for breakfast at the airport prior to boarding. I didn't want to eat anything too heavy but was happy that I was at a stage of my pregnancy where I can keep down some food. It was such a good feeling. Upon boarding I felt fine and fell asleep within the first 30 mins of our flight.

A few hours into the flight, I woke up with a weird feeling of lightheadedness. I tapped my boyfriend and told him I wasn't feeling well. I was in a middle seat with my boyfriend seated to my right in the aisle seat and a stranger sitting on the other side by the window.

Suddenly, the nausea came out of nowhere. Immediately it felt like I only had seconds before I was going to throw up!

"Oh no" I turned to my boyfriend and said. "I don't think I'm going to make it to the restroom." Oh God, please don't let me throw up on this stranger sitting next to me, I thought. Hold it in, just hold it in, I kept telling myself as my mouth filled with saliva.

My boyfriend took one look at me and knew it was about to go down. Or, I guess in this case, up. I was so afraid that I was going to vomit on an airplane full of passengers and couldn't imagine the stares and comments we were going to get.

Without saying a word, he quickly went into emergency mode. He reached forward and grabbed the barf bag in the seat pocket in front of him. In what seemed like one swift move, he handed me the bag, moved his body forward and leaned me over into his seat just in the nick of time for me to vomit in the bag behind his back. When I was done, he grabbed it from me, tied it up and placed it in the trash bag the stewardess was carrying down the aisle. Perfect timing. It was the smoothest move I've ever seen him do! No one, not even the passenger sitting on the other side of me reading his book with the overhead light on, had any clue that I had just thrown up inches away.

***W.I.D.E Tip: Try using Black Castor Oil to moisturize the skin on your stomach instead of lotion. I applied it vigorously twice a day during my entire pregnancy and never had one stretch mark. Maybe I was just lucky, but it's worth a try.***

# 8

# THE PRESSURE'S ON

Health wise, the remainder of our trip was pretty uneventful and for me that was a great thing. My next doctor's appointment was scheduled for that following week. Since I was feeling OK, as in not vomiting, no pains except for the occasional kicks to the crotch, I figured I'd go to this appointment alone. Usually, my boyfriend would take off from work to accompany me. Instead I left him behind and scheduled my appointment for mid-day. My doctor's office was only a short cab ride away from my job, so I casually made my way over around lunchtime.

Once there, the nurse took my vitals as usual and asked me how I was feeling. This was one of the rare times I replied that I was great. I had nothing to complain about. She began taking my blood pressure and made the strangest face. Saying nothing and me thinking nothing of it, she stopped and took it again. After the second time, she calmly looked at me and said "I'll be right back. I just need to grab your doctor."

When my doctor came in, he asked me how I was feeling, and again I replied, "I'm great." Now with just a hint of hesitation in my voice. I wasn't sure what was going on yet, but I knew that normally my doctor doesn't come into the examination room until after my vitals have been taken. So, sitting there with the blood pressure machine still attached to my arm, I knew something had to be wrong. He took my blood pressure again, himself. Now that for sure never happens.

"What's going on doc?" I questioned him curiously. That's when he told me my blood pressure was very high. I had a reading of 151/100 and said I needed to go to the hospital immediately. With utter confusion written across my face, he continued explaining to me that high blood pressure during pregnancy also referred to as **Gestational Hypertension,** may lead to an even more serious condition called **Preeclampsia.** My pressure was at a dangerously high level and he ordered that I go to the hospital for further evaluation.

You know what's funny, when he told me I needed to go to the hospital ASAP, I wasn't the slightest bit nervous. I didn't feel any sense of urgency because again to me, I felt totally fine. How was I going to explain having to leave work again this time to my boss? Just earlier that day I told him that I was feeling fine when he asked. What was I supposed to say now? As I gathered my things to leave the doctor's office, I figured that I'd go back to work first for a few hours, finish up some projects, then explain to my boss why I had to leave early, again.

I left the doctor's office and began hailing a taxi across the street. That's when one of the nurses came running out attempting to stop me.

"No!", she yelled out to me. "You can walk to the hospital from here. No need for a taxi. It's only a block or so away."

"I know", I replied to her while chuckling as I was very familiar by now with the location of the hospital. I explained to her that I was hailing a taxi as I planned on heading back to work first.

Her expression changed immediately and with a stern and serious voice she said "You really should go straight to the hospital. Your blood pressure is very high, and you need to be examined immediately." The intense look of concern on her face made it clear to me how serious this high blood pressure thing was and I turned and headed straight for the hospital.

On my short walk over, I called my boyfriend to let him know what was going on, even though I was still confused about it myself. "I don't get it. I feel fine." I told him. "I was expecting a normal doctor's visit today." No way did I think I would be heading back to my delivery hospital in the middle of the day.

Arriving at the hospital, I realized my doctor had called ahead as the staff was expecting me. I was greeted by the nurses and they escorted me in a wheelchair to the Labor and Delivery unit. A wheelchair, I thought? Was this necessary? Oh well, I'll just enjoy not having to be on my feet for a few minutes.

As I got undressed and changed into what was now becoming more like a uniform, a hospital gown that is; I thought to myself, this can't be that bad, can it? Aside from a little discomfort I wasn't experiencing any other symptoms. But there I was back at the hospital ready to be evaluated with no pain or vomiting and not realizing that I was in fact entering the most dangerous part of my pregnancy. I had no idea how serious high blood pressure especially during pregnancy could be. I was in for yet another surprise.

My exam showed no signs of protein in my urine and after a complete evaluation the doctors determined I had no signs of preeclampsia. I was relieved, but not out of the danger zone yet. My blood pressure was still very high, and the baby and I needed to continue being monitored. I had earned myself another stay at the hospital. This time, thank God, it was only for one night.

By the next day my blood pressure had gone back down to a normal reading and I was sent home. The doctors asked me to try my best to take in as much fluids as possible, as I was still very dehydrated. When he said it, I stopped for a second and realized I couldn't recall the last time I tried to have a drink of water. I knew water was important, but it wasn't until then that I realized without it, I was in danger of going into preterm labor. Still, I couldn't bring myself to drink it anyway. After the intense nausea it caused me throughout my pregnancy, I literally developed a mental block from wanting to drink any water at all.

The next day I followed up with a specialist referred by my doctor who dealt with high risk pregnancies. Together, they were hoping to figure out the best course of action for the remainder of my pregnancy. While meeting with the specialist, he explained that my blood pressure would need to be monitored with weekly office visits until I deliver. Weekly? All I thought about was how much more time that meant I would have to take off from work.

"Really doc? I have to come in to your office every week?" I asked. I didn't have many days off from work left and I was really hoping to save some for my maternity leave. I knew my health and that of my baby's should come first, and honestly it did. But it was beginning to feel like pregnancy and working just didn't mix. I was forced to go to work even when I could barely make it out of bed in the morning; and now even when the doctor was ordering me to take it easy, all I could think about was not being able to work. I just didn't have that luxury. It felt like a lose/lose situation.

I wish there was a way for expecting mothers like myself to just focus on staying healthy and growing these little humans inside of us, while not having to worry about throwing up on someone during a morning commute or getting kicked in the crotch by her fetus while in a meeting. Sigh, I thought. This sucks.

My pregnancy was turning out to be nothing at all like I had envisioned. I was drained, both physically and mentally. I flashed back to a day in my high school years. I was out shopping at the mall with my best friend when a pregnant woman walked into the department store. She was so beautiful. She wore a long fitted black maxi dress and had on a pair of laced up sandals. Her hair was pulled up into a neat bun and she complimented her look with a pair of large black sunglasses and red lipstick. She appeared to float through the perfume section in Macy's and my eyes followed her as though she was some sort of celebrity. "Wow, she's stunning" I told my friend. I remember thinking, that's exactly how I was going to look when I got pregnant. Chic and sexy. Boy was I wrong!

I was now a little over 7 months pregnant, not sleeping, barely eating, my belly looked and felt like an overstuffed sausage casing and I was still working full time. My job required that I be accessible 24/7 which of course, at times, can be very stressful. I was feeling totally defeated on the inside, but I had to force a smile on the outside. Why, you ask? Because I was pregnant, remember? And pregnancy is a blessing, right? I'm supposed to be delighted and smile every time someone sees me and says congratulations! After wanting to become a Mother for so long, how dare I complain and tell anyone this was the worse experience I've ever had? So, through my pale complexion, I would smile, say thank you, and carry on.

My commute became impossible. My daughter was still growing and with not having much room to move around, she was back to practicing the guitar with my urethra. My stomach felt so heavy that the shortest walk would leave me feeling exhausted and completely out of breath. Since I didn't have the option to work from home or to teleport myself there like Tabitha from Bewitched, my boyfriend arranged it so that I would have a ride to and from work every day. That made such a difference and alleviated some of the stress the commute was putting on my body.

My doctor had made it clear that placing me on bedrest would be the last resort. He explained that it may be more dangerous for me if I didn't continue being somewhat active; however, he also ordered that I try to remain as stress free as possible. Seriously? Does he even know me at all, I thought to myself? Does he you have any idea what my daily life consists of? The commuting? The level of stress I dealt with at work? The daily pain and discomfort I was feeling? Never being able to get more than 4 hours of sleep every night as I stayed up worrying about my high blood pressure? Then trying to calm myself down from worrying about my high blood pressure so that I didn't make it worse? Or realizing that I've maxed out my days off from work because I was hospitalized so often over the past several months. Let's not forget that I haven't purchased a single baby bottle, blanket or diaper yet for my baby and I had a gut feeling she would be making her grand entrance much sooner than anyone expects.

"Ha! Sure, Doc!" I told him. "I'll definitely try my best to remain stress free."

### ***TRANSITIONAL HYPERTENSION***
Also known as Gestational Hypertension or
Pregnancy-induced Hypertension

**Definition:** **New** onset of hypertension (**systolic ≥140 mmHg** and/or **diastolic ≥90 mmHg**) occurring **after 20 weeks gestation + no protein in the urine, edema (swelling) or end organ dysfunction.**

**Clinical Manifestations: usually not associated with symptoms.** If the blood pressure is high, it may cause headache or visual changes.

**Diagnostic Workup:** primarily to distinguish gestational hypertension from preeclampsia – urine protein, platelets, liver function tests & assessment of fetal status.

**Management: Supportive monitoring:** weekly blood pressure, urine protein, platelets & liver enzymes measurements. Ultrasound performed monthly to check for intrauterine growth restriction and weekly fetal nonstress testing in the third trimester.

• **Severe hypertension (≥160/110):** blood

pressure medications that are safe in pregnancy may be needed for some to reduce maternal stroke risk. Determined by your medical provider.

**When To Call Your Doctor:** Dizziness, headache or visual changes.

## *PREECLAMPSIA*

**Definition:**   **New** onset of high blood pressure (systolic ≥140 mmHg and/or diastolic ≥90 mmHg) occurring **after 20 weeks gestation + protein in the urine or end-organ dysfunction.**

**Clinical Manifestations:** May develop symptoms of end-organ damage - **cerebral or visual symptoms** (e.g., new-onset or persistent headaches, flashing lights, blurred vision), abdominal pain, decreased urine output, swelling of the extremities or fluid in the lungs.

• Mild: **≥140/90 mmHg + proteinuria ≥300mg** in a 24-hour urine specimen (or dipstick ≥1+).

• Severe: **≥160/110 mmHg + proteinuria ≥5g** in a 24-hour urine specimen (or dipstick ≥3+). Oliguria (<500ml of urine in 24 hours or 30cc/hour). Thrombocytopenia, **HELLP Syndrome:** **H**emolytic anemia **E**levated **L**iver enzymes and **L**ow **P**latelets.

• Sustained elevated blood pressure in pregnancy can lead to strokes or heart attacks in women and can compromise the fetus. **Women are also at the risk for developing eclampsia (preeclampsia + seizures or coma).**

**Management:** this should be closely discussed and determined by dialog with your medical care provider. Options include but are not limited to:

• Mild: ≥37 weeks gestation is best managed with delivery (but depending on the circumstances conservative management may be needed).

• Conservative: if < 34 weeks (daily weights, weekly blood pressure and dipstick, bed rest, antenatal corticosteroids to mature lungs if elective delivery is planned).

• Severe: prompt delivery is the definitive management after hospitalization + Magnesium sulfate to prevent seizures + blood pressure control with medications.

# 9

## DON'T LET ME BACK WITHOUT HER

After another long day of work, I remember coming home to find our bedroom filled with baby stuff. My boyfriend knowing how stressed out I was that our daughter may come early, took the initiative to go buy us what we needed. Normally that's a project I would have taken on myself. Unfortunately, I never felt well enough to handle a day of shopping.

Seeing boxes of diapers, wipes, bottles, wash rags, pacifiers, receiving blankets, onesies, socks, etc., gave me a sigh of relief. Even though I couldn't share in the shopping experience, I was glad at least that part was done. Of course, however, it also made me a little sad. I never would have imagined not having enough strength to go shopping for my own baby. I was so disappointed in what my road to becoming a first-time mom was turning into. I thought I would be one of those fashionable pregnant women who wore high heels right up until they were rolled into the delivery room. I wanted to look and feel as excited as I felt when I found out I was pregnant. But instead, there I was standing in my bedroom with tons of cute baby products that my boyfriend had to go pick out on his own.

Things didn't go as planned with work either. I thought I'd be able to work until my due date, but by my 8$^{th}$ month, my body couldn't handle the commute and long work days any longer. I went on maternity leave as of June 15$^{th}$, one month ahead of my scheduled due date. Saying goodbye to my coworkers, I went home that day hoping for a restful week as we were planning an extravagant baby shower for that Saturday.

I had a false labor alarm that week that turned out to only be Braxton Hicks contractions; however, seeing that the cramps weren't subsiding on their own, my doctor asked that I come in for a follow up. Given that I was now a little over 35 weeks with persistent high blood pressure, we didn't want to take any risks of me going into preterm labor.

"Look at her." I turned and said to my boyfriend while the specialist moved the sonogram probe over my belly. We both looked up and stared at the monitor. She looked so peaceful and oblivious to the fact that her mommy was in pain, not getting any sleep, had high blood pressure and was worrying about nearly everything under the sun. Instead, there she was resting so peacefully. It was amazing to see how resilient an unborn baby could be. After all the medications I've taken and the physical torment my body had gone through, it appeared as though nothing was affecting

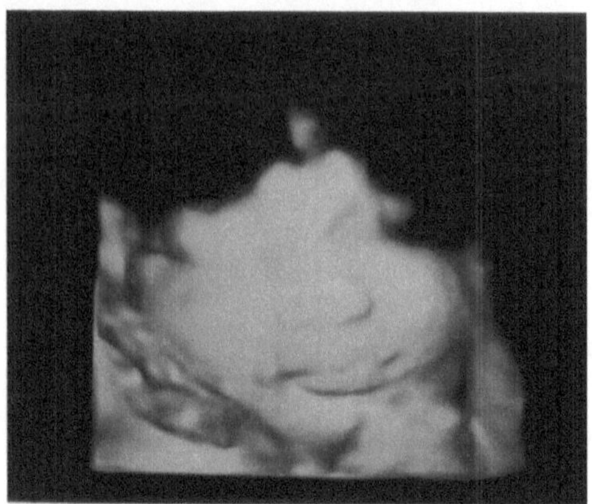

Sonogram image of my daughter at 35 weeks and 5 days gestation.

my baby in her warm cozy sac. I fell in love with her all over again. The sudden cramp in my stomach snapped my mind right back into reality.

Focus, I told myself. You must keep this baby in. She deserved every chance at a healthy, safe delivery and with everything I'd gone through, so did I.

Later that evening after getting home from the doctor's office, I laid on the couch to watch some TV and eat a slice of pizza, while my boyfriend went to bed early. Trying to take my mind off the pain I was still in, I realized what date it was. June 17th, the birthdate of one of my longest childhood girlfriends. I quickly reached for my phone to call and wish her a happy birthday before the day was over; while also hoping the friendly conversation would temporarily distract me from the pain.

I wished her a happy birthday and we chatted for about half an hour. The pain grew more and more intense. Not only was I feeling worse, but my stomach started looking completely distorted. As the cramps came on in waves across my stomach, it looked like my daughter was standing straight up riding them on a surfboard. I kept staring down at my stomach in disbelief that my body could even morph into such a weird shape. Not to mention that it felt like my uterus was being stretched to an unnatural size.

"You sure you're alright? You're not sounding too good over there" my friend asked. She must have heard my groans that I was trying to minimize on the other end of the phone. "You know, you still have time left to deliver her on my birthday" she teased.

Laughing, I replied "Nice try, but that's not happening."

Realizing I wasn't getting any relief laying on the couch, I ended our call and went to bed hoping to get some rest. I laugh at myself every time I think about this part. Rest? What made me think I could lay down and rest the pain away? How was I supposed to rest with my daughter practicing surfer moves in my uterus? What was I thinking trying to sleep it off? My belly looked like a mountain with 2 uneven peaks. The left side was Mount Everest and the right side was a ski slope for beginners.

"What are you doing in there?" I whispered to my daughter while cradling my belly. I had no idea what was going on inside of me.

I got in bed and tried to lay still. With every pain wave that came on, I grabbed a fist full of sheets with one hand and covered my mouth with the other trying my best not to scream. I didn't want to wake my boyfriend or scare him half to death while he was sleeping. At least one of us could get some rest. I felt my body starting to tense up and well, the scream happened anyway. He jumped out of bed and stared at me holding my belly.

"My stomach is doing something weird", I told him. "I think I need to go back to the hospital." He gave me that 'you can't be serious, we were just there' look. But as soon as I moved the covers to reveal my stomach, he took one look at our daughter's surfer-like moves and quickly said "Ok, let's go!"

I was having full blown contractions, but I still wasn't in active labor yet. I'll never forget the expression on the doctor's face while he examined me that night. He was down there, you know where, checking to see if I was dilating, when another contraction come on. My baby put on the same performance she had been gracing me with all night. It literally looked like she was standing straight up but just on the left side of my stomach. The doctor jumped so far back I thought he was going to fall!

"Whoa! What was that?" he asked.

"You tell me!" I replied while gripping onto both sides of the hospital bed. "She's been doing that for the past several hours."

With my heartrate increasing from the pain, the doctor started me on a dose of Morphine until it could be determined what was happening. God, more pain medicine, I thought? I wondered what sort of impact all of this was going to have on her. I felt like I was already failing at protecting my baby.

Snapping myself out of my thoughts, the doctor returned. This time accompanied by 4 other doctors. They each took turns introducing themselves and their specialties, but I couldn't hear anything over the sound of my heartbeat. There were now 5 doctors and 2 nurses in the room with us. All I kept thinking was this must really be bad to be drawing so much attention. Women go into labor every day. Do they all get this much attention?

Given the uncertainty of what was happening inside

of me, the doctors decided it was best for me to deliver immediately. Once my baby was delivered safely, they would then perform an exploratory surgery of my abdomen to try to determine the cause of my pain.

"Ok, then let's do it." I told them. I was ready. Ready to get her out of me and finally hold her. In my mind, I thought they were going to induce my labor in order to force my body to dilate, then I'd push my baby out and within a couple of days I'd be back home recovering. Well, if you've been following this story you can probably guess that with my luck, nothing with my pregnancy would be that simple.

First of all, I'd never get a chance to deliver naturally. They were instead prepping me for a C-Section. After safely delivering my baby, the doctor…

*W.I.D.E Tip: Wait, did I forget to mention that this was a completely new doctor whom I had only met that morning? Who I was now left to trust her to cut me open and deliver my child? Silly me, how could I forget that part?!*
*Where was my Specialist, you ask? The one I was referred to by my OBGYN? The one who was supposed to finish out the course of my pregnancy and safely deliver my baby? Well, turns out he was "not on call" that day. So, I was left to figure it out with a stranger.*
*Let that sink in for a moment, because, this happens far more often than you think. You try to plan out your pregnancy and delivery method as best as you can, and just when you think you have the perfect plan in place and you assume your doctor will be the one there with you, something like this happens. You're left to put*

*your life and your baby's life in the hands of a stranger.*
*My suggestion, make sure you and your partner, friend, family member or whomever you chose to be your advocate during your delivery, knows clearly what you want for you and for your baby. Make sure they know what your preferred delivery method is and to express that to the doctor as much as possible. Be sure to also have a second option should the first one become unavailable or unsafe. That person should also know what you want for your baby after delivery should you not be alert enough to provide the hospital staff with that information. What's your feeding plan? Is it OK for your baby to be given formula or do you only want him/her on breast milk? Do you want pain medication? These things may seem so obvious to you when you're not in an urgent situation but may become vital to your specific plan should you find yourself in an emergency.*
*Be sure to discuss all your options with your doctor well in advance and to share all that information with the person you've designated to be your advocate. But remember, be prepared for things to not go exactly as planned even with the best of pregnancies.*

Moving on… the doctor explained that after my C-Section, I would then be placed completely under anesthesia so that they may further perform an exploratory of my abdomen. You heard it right. I was to now undergo 2 surgeries back to back. Not exactly what I had in mind when we drove to the hospital at

1am that day.

My boyfriend and I sat still as the group of doctors explained the procedures to us. When they were done, I asked for a moment to speak with my boyfriend alone. As soon as what seemed like an entire medical class walked out of the room, I turned to face him realizing he had begun to tear up. Hearing what both procedures entailed along with the possible risks hit him harder than even he expected.

I stared him directly in his eyes and clearly said, "Don't let me back without her." I didn't care what might happen on that operating table, the option of me being alive in this world without my daughter was never to be an option. If there was ever a thought, even for a second should anything go wrong that there's an option between me or her, I needed him to make it crystal clear to everyone that there would be no option. Her life was the only choice. I was never more serious about something in my life. Realizing that my daughter was going to be delivered, then I would be put to sleep for more surgery, I needed to know that he would take over and would be her advocate and protect her life at all cost, while I was being operated on.

"Don't say that" he said as he interrupted me. But I quickly cut him off and demanded, "You better promise me. No other options." I repeated. With tears running down his cheeks, he said "I promise."

"Good", I replied "now, let's go meet our daughter."

# *10*

# THERE YOU ARE

Before I got pregnant, I would always say that there were no ifs ands or buts as to whether I would want an epidural for my labor. "They can give me 2 of them", I'd jokingly say to my friends. But boy, everyone forgot to tell me how uncomfortable they were to get. The doctors had me hunched over on a stretcher with my chin as close to my chest as I could get it. Remember, I was 8 months pregnant. Pregnant women can't bend over people! Our huge bellies make it kind of difficult. Anyway, they make you bend over as far as you can while sitting on the operating table, then they stick the longest needle I've ever seen inside your spine and they tell you not to move or else they may accidently hit a nerve that could leave you paralyzed. How was I supposed to do that?

"Try to stay still, please" the doctor said. "But, sir, you have a needle in my back." I replied. Everyone in the room laughed. I'm glad someone thought it was funny.

They numbed me up pretty good from the waist down as my boyfriend sat next to me on the non-fainting side of the curtain that was draped across my body at mid torso. Lying flat on my back with both arms strapped down on either side of me like Jesus on the cross, it felt like I was laying there for an eternity. But, the C-Section only took about 15 minutes.

My dream had finally come true. As the doctor pulled her from my womb, all I heard was my boyfriend's voice shout "She has your nose!" My eyes began searching the room to get a glimpse of my daughter for the first time. The nurses moved her over to a nearby table. Quickly, they asked my boyfriend to cut the umbilical cord. He had to hurry as the other end of the cord was still attached to the placenta inside of me. Oblivious to what was happening since I was tied down and couldn't move anything other than my head from left to right, I anxiously looked around the room still waiting to get a glimpse of my daughter.

Was everything OK, I wondered? "Where is she?" I asked impatiently. I couldn't hear or see her. That's when the nurse held up my little girl.

"She's perfect", I whispered as I stared at her. She didn't even cry. Her face looked like someone just woke her up from a nice nap and she was confused as to why it was suddenly so cold. I could not stop smiling. I wanted to jump off the operating table and hold her. Makes sense now why they had me strapped down.

"Count her fingers and toes", I said to my boyfriend. "Don't worry, they're all there" the nurse replied.

"Count them anyway, please", I asked him again. He did, and like the nurse said, they were all there. The nurse handed her to my boyfriend who then brought her over to me. I couldn't touch her as my hands were tied down. I just stared at her for a few seconds. My 6 lbs. 2 oz perfectly created baby. We didn't have much time as the doctors had already began prepping for my second surgery.

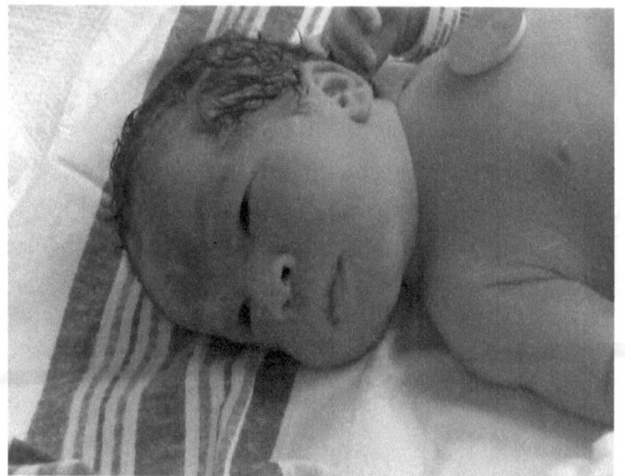

**Isabelle at only 10 minutes old.**

I whispered in her ear "Mommy will be right back, Isabelle. I love you. Thank you for letting me be your Mommy."

I looked up at my boyfriend. "Please, don't let her out of your sight", I asked him as I slowly drifted into total sedation. I breathed a sigh of relief knowing she made it out safely. I did it.

Several hours later I woke up in the recovery unit in excruciating pain. Quickly, the nurse standing next to my bedside began administering pain medication for relief. Thank God. Our friends and family soon gathered around me. As the pain meds started to kick in so did extreme fatigue. In between all the hugs and kisses I was receiving, I realized it was Thursday and our baby shower was supposed to be in 2 days! I sent an unexpected birth notification text to everyone invited to our baby shower, postponing the event to what would now be a welcoming party. I probably should have let someone else handle that task since I had just given birth and was still high as a kite on meds. But hey, that's the control freak in me.

My boyfriend walked into the room and I realized he had kept his promise to me and had stayed by our daughter's side the entire time I was in surgery. He told me she was placed in the Neonatal Intensive Care Unit (NICU). She was doing well, but since she was born at only 35 weeks and 6 days, she was considered a late term preemie. Which meant her tiny lungs and other organs needed to be monitored to confirm they were functioning properly. With sleep rapidly creeping up, I decided to use this time to get some well-deserved rest.

Nearly 30 hours had passed before I was finally able to hold my daughter for the first time. We were kept on different floors and after undergoing back to back surgeries, my body needed time to recover. My boyfriend rolled me over in a wheelchair to the NICU while still hooked up to an epidural and an IV line. I couldn't walk yet. The epidural kept my lower half completely numbed. The nurse placed my daughter in my arms and I held her up against my chest closely.

Taking in the moment, I smelled her hair and caressed her cheek with my fingers. It was almost as though she recognized my touch even though I've never held her until that moment. Wanting confirmation that it was in fact her mommy, my one-day old baby wobbled and lifted her tiny little head all on her own to look up at me. She opened her eyes and searched my face for confirmation. Her gaze was priceless. It was almost as though her eyes were saying, "There you are, Mommy. You finally came back." Then, she wobbled her head over to the direction of my nipple and latched on.

It was amazing. Even the nurse was surprised. "It's like she was waiting for you", she said. "I've never seen a newborn lift her head on her own before."

That moment, everything, and I mean everything I went through, was worth it. I was holding my perfect little baby girl and I was now forever, a Mother.

We stayed in the hospital for 4 days before being released. Those days were not without their own set of adventures. On my third day in the hospital, the epidural was finally removed. I began feeling pain yet again in my stomach. I remember thinking the pain must be from my 2 surgeries. The exploratory procedure the doctors performed showed that part of my intestine had been hooked on to a fibroid in my uterus. I guess that would explain the pain I felt. Perhaps my body was just still recovering and that's why I was in pain again? With my pain level steadily increasing by the hour, I asked a nurse to please send in a doctor.

The doctor looked at me in confusion as she didn't understand why I would still be in so much pain. Upon examining me, she also realized my lower abdomen where I was feeling the most discomfort, was very sensitive to touch.

"When was the last time you peed?" she asked. As though she asked me a complicated biology question, I realized I had no idea when the last time was that I peed on my own. The catheter used during my surgery was removed immediately afterwards; however, the epidural was not. It was left in order to manage my pain. What no one seemed to remember was that although the epidural was keeping my lower body totally numbed from pain, it also numbed the feeling or urge to pee even though my bladder was completely full!

The pain was from the tension placed on the lining of my bladder as it expanded like a balloon. We all know what happens when a balloon gets filled with too much air, right? Well, the same thing happens to a bladder when it's filled with urine as well! Quickly signaling for the nurse to bring her a pitcher, the doctor told me that she was going to have to insert another catheter immediately to alleviate the pressure on my bladder.

I felt I needed to remind her that I'm still very much awake. "Ma'am, don't you think you should put me out again for that?" I asked while holding my stomach and cringing in pain. She tried her best to calm me down and explained that being put under anesthesia was completely unnecessary and if I allowed her to do this right now, I would be feeling better within minutes.

I mean, I knew her putting me to sleep wasn't necessary, I was just hoping she would knock me out anyway! Who wants to be wide awake while they stick a tube into their bladder? Was she not aware of the dance parties my daughter was having on my urethra when I was pregnant? My poor urethra, I thought. Hasn't it been through enough?

But there was no time to lay there and feel sorry for myself. This needed to be done and it needed to be done now. Kicking everyone except for the nurse out of the room, the doctor inserted a catheter into my bladder. Oh boy! The amount of urine that came out of me was insane! She had to have the nurse grab a second pitcher because the first one filled up so quickly.

"Wow!", the doctor said in amazement. "You had almost 2 liters in there." Thank goodness that was over. The relief came immediately.

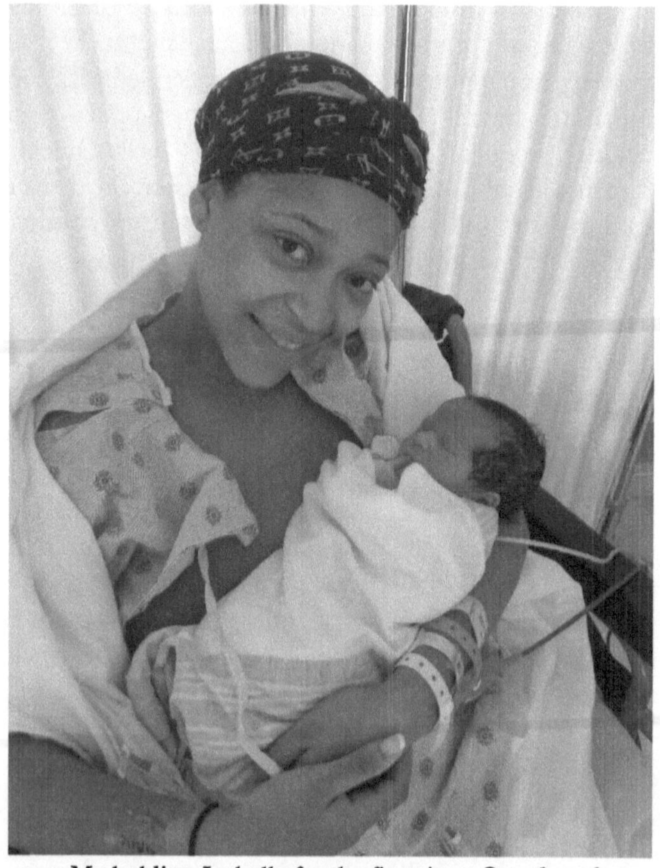

**Me holding Isabelle for the first time. One day after delivery.**

# 11

# MOTHERHOOD

After having such a difficult pregnancy, you would think that I would have lots to complain about with motherhood. After all, that's when the sleepless nights, late night feedings, gassy, crying, colicky baby part kicks in, right? Well, not this mommy. No complaints from me! Because although I was going through all the standard newborn baby drama, I was literally so in love with her and with motherhood in general, that it made everything feel better.

I mean yes, of course it was rough in the beginning. The breastfeeding, the pumping - of which I am proud to say that I quit after trying for 2 months. It was just too hard for me. I was placing my breasts inside of a machine that had a suction cup at the end of it and it made me feel like it was sucking my entire chest in through a tiny tube. Ouch! No, thanks. It felt like I was abusing my boobs. But hey, if you can do it, more power to you sister! Keep up the great work; however, this momma gracefully bowed out after 2 months and

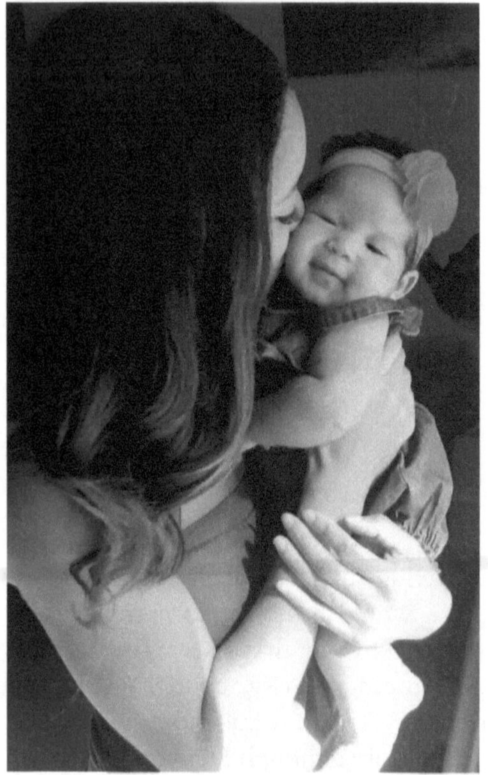

**Me and Isabelle, at 3 months old.**

started my daughter on formula. Don't get me wrong, I believe breastmilk is best; so, if you're able to, do it. But if you can't, don't let anyone make you feel guilty about it.

The months passed quickly, and I tried to spend every second I could with my daughter before going back to work. Things had changed now that I was someone's Mother. The way I viewed life and my priorities had all changed. Nothing came before the health and happiness of my daughter. Everything changed now that I was a Mom, including my body.

Since I was rarely able to keep any food down, I only gained a total of 19 pounds during my pregnancy. Half of that was water weight and my daughter took up another 6 pounds. That means I barely gained anything at all. Although that might sound appealing to some, given my circumstances, it made for an unhealthy situation.

I lost the water weight very quickly but even though I could eat, I was thinner than I was before getting pregnant. When I went back to work in 3 months, my coworkers would compliment me on how great they thought I looked. "Thanks, but I think I could definitely use a few pounds" I would respond. I didn't like how thin I was because it made me feel unhealthy. Personally, I didn't like feeling like a sudden gust of wind could blow me away. It wasn't about how I looked as much as it was how I felt. I just wanted to *feel* healthy again. It took my body a very long time to recover from pregnancy.

Having a baby takes a major toll on a woman's body. Even in the best of pregnancies, your body needs time to heal itself. So, if your pregnancy wasn't a walk in the park, it's natural that it may take longer for most things to get back to normal. I say most because there are some things that will never be the same again ladies. But guess what? That's OK too! We need to learn to wear our pregnancy scars with pride. Think about it. Our bodies go through an incredible transformation so that we may create life. Your scars are like a badge of honor for doing what only YOU could do. Don't be too hard on yourself. You just created a HUMAN.

I laugh in disbelief every time I think about what my body was able to create. Did I just make a whole human being? It's so crazy. No wonder why women feel like we have super powers after giving birth. It's because we really are incredible super beings. Think about it; I was so miserable during my pregnancy. But regardless of how I felt, my body still knew exactly what to do all on its own to create life. Then once that life was created, my body produced the nutrition it needed to grow, again all on its own. Wow, incredible indeed.

As incredible as it was to know that my body could create life, I hated every time someone asked me "So, when are you having your next baby?" Were they crazy? "Never again!" I'd respond. There's no way in hell I was ever going through that again.

# *12*

## WHAT? YOU'RE WHAT?!

Getting back in the swing of things took time. It had been a year and a half since giving birth and I still felt like my body was recovering from the 8 months of trauma it had endured. But I wasn't complaining. I was feeling good and although the recovery was slow, I was finally beginning to feel like myself again.

Every December we held a Christmas party at our home. We would invite all our close friends and family and have a seriously good time. Plenty of food and drinks to go around for everyone. After having my daughter, I pretty much stopped drinking alcohol all together, so the drinking part I left to our guests. No, not because I was breastfeeding (I gave that up remember? Proud quitter over here), instead it was because I was so afraid of getting a hangover. It reminded me so much of the nausea I had when I was pregnant, that the thought of having a glass of wine grossed me out. Before having my daughter, I would love enjoying a glass of wine with dinner. Especially after a long, stressful day of work. But now, things were different. My friends all thought I was crazy. I would too if I had an easy pregnancy.

Anyway, back to our Christmas party. I've always loved throwing events. It brings me joy to see everyone enjoying themselves, eating, drinking, laughing and creating priceless moments together. To ensure just that, I would personally do all the prep work for the parties myself. The cooking, set up, decor, everything needed to ensure a great time would be had by everyone in attendance. This year would be no different. I spent a week preparing for our holiday party and it was a hit. With all the work it took to execute a successful event, I thought it was no wonder why I felt so exhausted afterwards.

The day after our party I stayed in all day recovering. Normally, recovering meant just staying home, spending time with my daughter who was now a very active, crawling baby, doing some light housework and just taking it easy. But on this recovery day, it seemed all I could do was sleep. Good thing it was a Sunday and my boyfriend was home. He took care of our daughter while I slept most of the day.

What was even more bazaar was the fact that I was still so tired 2 days after our party, that I had to call out of work. I stayed home that Monday but sleep, even though I was exhausted, wasn't an option this time. Since I was staying home, of course I kept my daughter home with me instead of us sending her to daycare. I felt like I barely had enough time with her in my opinion anyway since I was back to work full-time. That meant I was back to being out of the house 12 hours **a day**. So even though I was very tired, I kept her home and we had a great day together.

Watching her play I remember thinking how quickly she was growing up. It seemed like just yesterday she was in my tummy. I stared at her and tried my best to take in that moment. She was just smiling away while drool ran down her cheeks. Seasoned mothers always told me the time would go by quickly and it sure was. I was glad I stayed home that day. I would spend every moment of every day with her, if I could.

The week continued to be a struggle for me. Staying awake that is. Why was I so tired? At first, I thought maybe I was coming down with something because the exhaustion would seem to hit me like a truck. But with no fever or any signs of a cold, I had to figure out what could be making me so tired.

That Friday afternoon while on the phone at work with a client, we were discussing dates to have a meeting prior to the New Year. That's when I suddenly realized it was almost the end of the month. Wait, I thought to myself, did I have my period yet this month? Now before having my daughter, I would experience severe cramps and very heavy bleeding with my menstrual cycle. So, there was never a time when I forgot if my period came already or not. It was one of those things that you just wouldn't forget because you were happy when it was finally over for that month and already dreaded having it again the next. But after having my daughter, my period returned 3 months later but now they were very light. Most months I only bled for a couple of days and spotted for another day or two. As opposed to the 6 days of heaving bleeding I used to have before. Even my cramps were gone. Aside from having my beautiful daughter, an easier period was the one good thing that pregnancy gave me.

Staring at my calendar, I realized I had missed my

period. AHHHHH! Remember my little trick I talked about at the beginning of my story. I gave that up. Something about tricking yourself for years then having the joke be on you, forces you to give up the shenanigans. I was fresh out of tricks for making my period come. Besides, once you've become a mom, you just know when you're pregnant again. Sitting at my desk now with a blank stare and not even realizing I was still on the phone with a client, I knew why I'd been feeling like I hit a brick wall all week. I was pregnant, *again*.

Snapping myself out of a self-induced hypnotized state, I finally hung up with my client and quickly made my way down to the pharmacy and picked up a pregnancy test. As if I even needed it. I think somewhere in the back of my mind I was holding onto a slither of hope that I wasn't what I thought I was even though I already knew I was. You know what I mean? Less than a minute after taking the test, it was once again confirmed.

Want to know what went through my head? It went something like this… Oh my God, oh my God, oh my God, oh my God… Yeah, that pretty much sums up my reaction.

I left the bathroom, grabbed my cellphone and headed outside my office to call my now, fiancé. I was eager to share the news with him. Not out of excitement but mostly, confusion. I mean, obviously I knew *how* this happened, but I didn't have a clue how to feel about it.

Our call went as I expected. He was home with our daughter, so I could hear her in the background yelling, laughing and crying all at the same time. Trying my best to speak over her background noise without shouting my news to everyone walking by, I told him we were pregnant, again. As soon as I uttered the words out loud, something hit me. A strange vibe of confidence. I think I could do this, I thought to myself.

Well, something must have hit my fiancé on the other end too, but it wasn't the same emotion that I had suddenly felt. He remained completely silent.

"Hello?" I said several times. I could still hear our daughter in the background laughing, so at least I knew she was OK. But there was complete radio silence from my him. "Did you just die on me?" I asked. "You'd better not be dead over there." I said.

"No", he replied. "I'm still here." Finally, a response. I guess fell he into a self-induced hypnotized state too. I knew the feeling.

"So, what do you think?", I asked. "OK", he replied.

"What? OK? Just OK?! You can't be serious." I said to him. I started to get angry but then I realized, what in the world did I expect him to say? Was he supposed to be as excited as he was before when I told him I was pregnant with our daughter? Was he supposed to be upset? Nervous? I realized I was waiting for his reaction so that I could determine how *I* felt, and that wasn't fair of me to do. The man was probably afraid to show any reaction. Afterall, I did just call him in the middle of the day while he was feeding our daughter to tell him that we were about to go through another pregnancy. As I thought about it, I should have probably waited to tell him when I got home that night. We got off the phone and I tried to continue my day hiding the fear that was slowly creeping up of what was in store again for my body.

The next day I called my OBGYN to share the news

and schedule an appointment. As the days went on, my fear became less and less. My fear didn't come from the fact that we were going to have another baby. Secretly, I wanted another baby. I wanted my daughter to have a sibling close in age that she can grow up with. I wanted for her the sibling relationship I have with my brothers. Although I was the youngest, which meant I was the one always getting beat up, I loved having brothers that I could turn to when I needed them. I felt a sense of protection having them around. I didn't want my daughter to be alone.

What I was afraid of was the process of having another baby. I wasn't sure if my body was able to handle that trauma again. I felt like I was still healing, and I was honestly petrified of what another pregnancy was going to do to me.

Putting those fears aside, I was ready to ride it out. At my doctor's appointment, we determined that I was approximately 5 weeks along and we scheduled my following appointment for a month and a half later. I expressed my concerns to my doctor and he comforted me by explaining that every pregnancy is different, and that one horrible pregnancy experience didn't mean that I was doomed to experience another one this time.

Maybe he was right, I thought to myself. Afterall, I was honestly feeling great. I mean I had a great appetite, I wasn't feeling as tired as I was last week, there was no nausea at all and to top it off, my skin looked amazing! In fact, I think it was glowing! Yes! I can actually glow during pregnancy! Woohoo! I felt so encouraged after my visit that I just couldn't stop smiling. "I can do this" I told myself. This time it was going to be different.

Now excited to share the news, I called my mom later that evening. I wish I could say she was as excited to hear the news as I was to tell her. Her reaction, like that of my fiancé's, was quite different than the first time.

"What?! she exclaimed on the other end of my cell phone. "You're what? What did you just say?!" she asked again. But it wasn't anger I heard in her voice, it was fear. Now I understood the reason behind my fiancé's radio silence when I shared the news with him. It was fear. I get it. Here are the 2 people who experienced what I went through first hand when I was pregnant with my daughter. My fiancé especially saw the daily toll it took on my body. My mother, although she was a distance away, would call me every day when I was pregnant to ask how I was doing, and I could hear the pain in her voice when she spoke to me. Her voice was full of helplessness. Her daughter was suffering almost every day and there was nothing she could do to help me. My mother had a very different experience with pregnancy than I had, so she never knew what to say or what she could do to help me. That alone had to be so hard for her. Watching her only daughter suffer, day after day for months. It made sense why her reaction to this pregnancy came off a bit harsh.

"I can do it, Mom", I assured her. "I feel great. I'm not nauseous or anything. I've actually been eating a lot", I told her. "Everyone says that each pregnancy is different. This one was going to be different than before. You'll see, Mom. Don't worry." I tried my best to reassure her.

"I've got to go." she replied with sadness in her voice. Somehow, I knew she was getting off the phone with me to cry. Not the reaction I had hoped for to say the least. But as a mother myself now, I understood it.

The next several days were great. I woke up every morning fearing today would be the day I would awaken to nausea; but thankfully I didn't. I enjoyed every moment of it. The New Year had come along, and I felt in my heart it would be a great year for me, for us, for our family. My fiancé started getting a little excited himself about the idea of having another baby in the house. We'd talk about how much of a great big sister our daughter was going to be.

I began doing all the things I didn't think of doing my first pregnancy. I know I was still very early, but I vowed I would use this time to plan properly. Something my health never gave me the opportunity to do before. While at a friend's birthday party that weekend, we shared our exciting news. Even that was something I would have normally waited a few months to do. But honestly, I just couldn't contain my excitement. We talked amongst us what life would be like with more than one child. I asked my friends who had more than one child a ton of random questions. Like what kind of stroller should we get? I guess we'll also need another crib, right? Will the new baby break the great sleep routine that we've now finally mastered with our daughter? My questions just kept coming but you could hear the excitement in my voice. Finally, I thought to myself, finally pregnancy was going to be wonderful.

# 13

# DETERMINATION

Week 7: I remember waking up in the middle of the night to get a cup of water. It was a cold, January night so the heat in our home was on keeping us and especially our daughter nice and warm; however, the heat also made my throat dry. I crawled out of bed slowly not to wake up my fiancé or our daughter who was fast asleep in her crib and made my way to the kitchen. I drank a full glass of water, stopped for a second to pet our dog and started making my way back to bed. My eyes were barely open as I walked back into the bedroom.

As I started to creep back into bed, my eyes flew open. Oh no, oh no! Knowing what I was feeling all too well, I rushed to the bathroom and the water I literally just drank came right back up. My heart was racing. It can't be. I felt great just yesterday. I was just fine even a minute ago. My heartbeat got so loud it was like someone was playing it over a loudspeaker in the bathroom. This cannot be happening again, I thought to myself as fear surged through my body as I stared at myself in the mirror. I could feel my pulse beating through every vein in my body. It was like I was having a nightmare and I couldn't wake myself up from it.

I walked back into the bedroom and realized everyone was still sleeping. Good, I thought for sure my episode had woken them. I slowly got back into bed, laid my head on my pillow and pulled the covers over me. Like a scared child who had a monster living under her bed, that no one else could see, hear, or feel. I realized my scary monster had come back to haunt me yet again. I closed my eyes knowing it was there with me and a tear fell down my face onto my pillow. My monster, nausea, was back.

The next day I immediately took action. I wasn't about to let this destroy my pregnancy experience again. I called my doctor and told him I was already having nausea and vomiting and wanted to get on medication to alleviate it immediately. I didn't want to wait it out like I did the last time only to suffer. I couldn't take the chance this time around. I had a one-year old baby that needed her mother to take care of her. There was no time to wait and see if it would just go away.

Having already thrown up again that morning while getting ready for work, I made it clear to my doctor that I did not want the same pregnancy experience I had before. I still had nausea medication from my previous pregnancy but wasn't sure if they were still OK to take. Yes, the ones that worked for a week then stopped. I still had them in my medicine cabinet. I thought if I started them early enough this time, things would be different. After confirming the date on my prescription bottle with my doctor, he said they were still OK to take. Immediately I took one.

Now at work hours later, I realized I was still very nauseous. I realize this time was different than before. Not only did my nausea come on earlier, but it was even more intense. At least before there was a weaning in period. Remember when I threw up for the first time while pregnant with my daughter and I thought the queasiness was cute? Yeah, well there was nothing cute about it this time. I went from feeling perfectly fine to full blown nausea and constant vomiting. Still, I was determined to have a different experience this time.

I asked another co-worker who had recently had a baby what she took to help with her nausea. Of course, I didn't say it was for me. Although I was starting to share the news with a handful of friends, I was nowhere near ready to share the news with anyone at work. Instead, I told my co-worker that I had a friend who was going through a difficult bout of nausea and vomiting with her pregnancy; and that since mine was so horrible before, I didn't know what to suggest for her to ask her doctor about taking.

Diclegis, she replied was the name of the anti-nausea medication she was prescribed during her pregnancy. "Thanks!", I told her. I'll let my *friend* know.

I gave the Ondansetron a few days to see if they would kick in and alleviate my nausea. When it didn't work, I called my doctor and asked him to prescribe me Diclegis. I was hopeful that this drug would work better for me. The way my co-worker explained how it did wonders for her, I just knew it would make me feel better. At that point I was almost 8 weeks and was already throwing up daily. At least 2 to 3 times a day. God, I thought, pregnancy really hates me. The nausea was constant.  It literally never went away. It felt like a permanent horrible hangover.

Making it into work was hard enough the first time around when I only had to worry about taking care of myself. Now try to imagine having to take care of a one year old and going to work full time while feeling like this. I was determined to make myself better. I didn't have a choice really. Where perhaps I had the option of taking a few days off from work, I didn't have the option of taking a minute off from motherhood. How was I going to explain to my daughter that her mommy couldn't feed her right now because she was too busy throwing up?

I immediately called the pharmacy once I knew my prescription had been called in. I didn't want to waste a minute picking it up once it was ready. The response I received from the Pharmacist when I called totally pissed me off. She told me that my insurance company wouldn't authorize my prescription.

"What?", I asked her as if she was speaking to me in a foreign language. "What do you mean they won't authorize it?" She suggested I call my insurance company to discuss the authorization process with them.

I hung up with (probably on) her and grabbed my insurance card to call the number on the back. Apparently, there's a whole authorization process that you must go through before your insurance company will agree to pay for certain medications. Funny, I thought. I didn't need an authorization for the pain pills they prescribed me during my last pregnancy. But now, there I was laying in bed, a spit bucket next to me because not only couldn't I control when I threw up, I also couldn't control the amount of saliva building up in my mouth every 5 minutes. With all that, now I had to also be on the phone with my insurance company that I pay every month for health coverage and debate with them why I needed my prescription filled asap. After being transferred at least 4 times, finally, I got a somewhat competent representative who explained the authorization process.

First, my doctor would need to complete a request form explaining the need for the medication. I guess just a prescription wasn't enough this time. Frustrated, aggravated and spitting into a bucket every few minutes, I hung up with my insurance company and called my doctor's office again. The receptionist assured me she would get on it right away and would send the requested information.

I gave it an hour or so before following up. That gave me enough time to go throw up, for the 3rd time that day. I'm glad I had decided to take the day off. My fiancé was at work and we sent our daughter to daycare since I was feeling so miserable. I knew this was the only day I had to get this prescription and hopefully get myself back on the road to feeling better and having a healthy pregnancy.

Confirming the requested info was sent in, the next step was to follow up with my insurance company. The reps response pissed me off yet again. Do they like making pregnant people mad? She told me that the person assigned to handle my request was "out to lunch".

"I'm sorry ma'am, did you say she was out to lunch? Oh, well lucky her." I replied. "She's out eating. That must be nice. I wouldn't know anything about that because you see, I can't hold down *anything*. When I try to eat, I throw up. Do you know what that means?" I asked her. Not waiting for her to respond, I continued my rant "It means that neither I or the baby that I'm growing inside of me is able to get any nutrition! Hence why I need this prescription, ma'am. But I see that that can't happen right now because the representative that's supposed to be helping me is out enjoying her life."

Taking a pause from my emotional pregnant lady meltdown, there were a few seconds of silence. The now probably petrified representative on the line finally replied, "Let me try to help you."

"Oh, thank you", I said. "What was your name again?" I asked. She told me, and I pretended to listen and care. "Thank you again", I said. "I truly appreciate it."

We had a brief 3-way conference call with my doctor's office to ask a list of ridiculous questions such as, "Why does she need this medication? Have you tried anything else? On a scale from 1-10, how bad is her nausea?" Are you freaking kidding me? I thought to myself. Is she really asking these questions?

I interrupted the rep and asked, "Do you think this is a joke? I'm literally throwing up so much every day that most of the time there isn't even anything inside of me to throw up! I have a one-year old baby that I can barely muster up the strength to hold because I'm so weak and you're on the phone trying to find a reason to deny me from getting the help I need? Do you know what it feels like to be nauseous even while you're asleep? Or what it's like not wanting to even get out of bed every morning knowing what the day had in store for you? But you have no choice because you're a mother and there's an innocent little life that you've already created that's counting on you to take care of her. Even as I'm talking to you right now, I'm swallowing my saliva every 10 seconds knowing that I'm going to throw up again!"

I guess she got the point that time. She immediately approved my prescription and an hour later, it was ready for pick up at the pharmacy.

# 14

## TRISTAN & YSEULT

My first day on Diclegis went well. The nausea wasn't gone completely, but I felt some relief. Enough that I could get up in the morning, get my daughter ready for daycare, get myself ready for work and make it there with no accidents on the train. At least I wasn't throwing up I thought to myself. Still, I didn't feel quite right. Taking the feeling for what it was and accepting that I was in for another complicated pregnancy, I carried on with my day keeping my feelings to myself. Work would at least give me a temporary distraction.

The next day I could feel the nausea creeping back. I had taken 2 pills at bedtime the night before, as directed. It worked for me yesterday, so I wasn't sure why today was different. After having lunch at work, I threw up. Trying not to feel too discouraged about it, I thought maybe my lunch was too heavy and I should stick to bland foods. I called my doctor for any ideas. He suggested I'd take one tablet in the morning and the other at night instead of both at once. Since the medication was in a slow release form, perhaps having it in my body on a more consistent basis would help. I started the new dose right away.

Several hours later I was home and getting ready to have dinner. The nausea hadn't let up yet, but I was determined to keep some food down. I didn't make it home from work until 8pm every day, so my time with my daughter was always limited. The short time I was able to spend with her was very important to me. That evening while giving her a bottle, I started taking in spoonful's of chicken noodle soup I had prepared for myself. Every sip was a challenge. I was trying very hard to convince myself that this soup wasn't going to come right back up.

Determined to give my growing fetus some nutrients, I finished my soup and sat back on the couch very still with my daughter in my arms. Concentrate, I kept telling myself. I closed my eyes trying to focus on not throwing up. I held it in for as long as I could.

Almost an hour later I got up, put my daughter who had fallen asleep in my arms down in her crib and headed straight to the bathroom sink. Barely making it there, it felt like the food hadn't digested at all as it came back up. If you've ever thrown up before you know how not only gross it is but how exhausting the task can be on your body. Imagine having to deal with that every day, several times a day, non-stop. At least when you throw up from a hangover you start feeling better. Not with this. What is this really, I asked myself? It felt a million times worse than the symptoms described as morning sickness.

As I rinsed my face off from the tears scrolling down my cheeks, I looked down to see the Diclegis pill I had taken hours ago now in my bathroom sink. I couldn't believe it. The medicine I was taking to make me feel better was still in my stomach and I threw it up, whole.

That's when the depression began. What now? Feeling completely defeated again and disappointment, I walked out of the bathroom and just went to bed. Lying there staring into the darkness I remember thinking just how inadequate of a woman I must be that my body couldn't even handle pregnancy. The one thing it was clearly created to be able to do. I fell asleep crying into my pillow, trying not to wake up my daughter.

The days passed, and my nausea and vomiting had gotten worse. I was now vomiting constantly almost every hour. The most I'd counted was 12 times in one day. Working became impossible. How was I supposed to explain getting up from my desk every hour to head to the ladies room? A weak bladder, maybe? That's a good enough excuse. I think I'll go with that should anyone ask me.

I was barely eating anything and when I did, I tried holding it down as long as I could so that my baby could absorb some nutrition. What must my baby be going through in there? I was only 8 weeks along and I already felt my body deteriorating. Again, I couldn't hold down water at all. How badly is all of this affecting my unborn child?

One day during one of my trips to the bathroom, after throwing up I looked down in the toilet before flushing and I was shocked to see traces of blood. It was very easy to detect since I only threw up bile. Oh my God. Now I'm throwing up blood? What the hell was going on with me. Sadly, it didn't only happen that one time. I continued to throw up blood almost every time from that point on.

I started researching my symptoms in depth, but nothing I found felt familiar to what I was experiencing. Yes, they mentioned the nausea and perhaps some vomiting may occur with regular morning sickness, but it wasn't to the extreme measures of what I had going on with me.

Finally, I came across a term that validated what I was going through. Extreme cases of morning sickness known as **Hyperemesis Gravidarum (HG),** feels very different from regular morning sickness. While most women who experience morning sickness can tolerate its symptoms, those of us with HG have symptoms that are so intense that they cause a major impact on our day to day lives.

Finally, something that made sense. I could finally place a name to how I've been feeling. I guess I wasn't the only one who's gone through this, I remember thinking to myself. So now what? Most women who have experienced HG during pregnancy are more likely to experience it again with every pregnancy. So much for every pregnancy being different, huh. That makes sense since I was just as miserable when I was pregnant with my daughter as I was now. But this time, it's happening earlier and seemed to be even more intense.

***W.I.D.E Tip:*** *If you're confused or having difficulty determining whether you're experiencing morning sickness versus HG, you may find the following comparison chart helpful. Together with your doctor, you can determine how to alleviate your discomfort.*

| MORNING SICKNESS | HYPEREMESIS GRAVIDARUM |
|---|---|
| • Nausea and/or vomiting usually lasting **up until 16 weeks gestational age (most common in the first trimester).** | • More severe form of morning sickness |
| <u>Symptoms:</u> mild nausea and/or vomiting that does not usually interfere with your ability to eat or drink or your ability to function (although it can often cause discomfort and some disruption to a daily routine).<br>• Usually not associated with vomiting bile or blood.<br>• The nausea is usually episodic with infrequent vomiting.<br>Usually not associated with weight loss (if weight loss occurs, it is usually minimal). | <u>Symptoms:</u> **severe or constant nausea and/or vomiting** that often **interferes with your ability to eat or drink throughout the day and/or the ability to function (may not be able to work due to symptoms, fatigue or weakness).**<br>• Vomiting may be so severe that it can contain bile or blood.<br>• The nausea can be continuous with frequent vomiting.<br>Usually **associated with weight loss** of ≥5% of pre-pregnant weight, dehydration and electrolyte imbalance. It can cause other blood disturbances |
| <u>Treatment</u><br>• Dietary and lifestyle changes<br>Anti-nausea medications | <u>Treatment</u><br>• Similar to morning sickness but **may require additional IV hydration and electrolyte replacement.** Severe cases may need calorie replacement intravenously. |
| <u>Prognosis:</u> usually resolved by 16 weeks gestational age with gradual improvement but occasional nausea or vomiting may occur during the remainder of pregnancy. | <u>Prognosis:</u> may persist after 16 weeks gestational age with nausea and or vomiting that may occur during the remainder of pregnancy. Patients may need help caring for themselves due to severe symptoms & inability to function. |

I shared with my fiancé that I had vomited blood earlier that day. His face was a look of shock, but he also didn't appear to be too surprised. It's like he was waiting for things to get worse, but also hoped it wouldn't happen this time.

"You OK?", he asked. "No", I replied staring down at the floor as my eyes filled with tears. "I don't think I'm going to ever be OK."

I walked into the bedroom, kissed my daughter who thankfully had already fallen asleep since I didn't have the energy to stay up with her, and I went straight to bed. While falling asleep for the first time the thought crossed my mind, what if I don't make it? What if my body couldn't see this pregnancy through to the end? Can my unborn baby survive what my body was enduring? If I didn't make it, what would happen to my daughter? The thought of not being around to raise my daughter scared me so much that I forced myself to sleep, just so that I could stop thinking about it.

For the first time, I considered terminating my pregnancy. Not wanting to do it, I thought if I watched enough videos about abortions, I could scare myself into no longer considering it as an option. Maybe in turn I would gain some much-needed strength to keep pushing. It was kind of like a new trick I was playing on myself. Anytime I thought I couldn't do it anymore or felt like my body was giving out on me, I would get on the internet and look up pregnancy terminations. I tortured myself with images and graphic videos of what happens during a termination. It would scare me so much that mentally, I convinced myself each time to try to hang on. You could do this, I would tell myself after every time I threw up. My trick worked, for a while.

It was a Saturday afternoon in February and I was home alone with my daughter. By now it was a struggle to do just about anything, but this day seemed exceptionally hard. I was 9 weeks pregnant and before getting out of bed in the morning, I would have to plan out how I was going to take care of my daughter. I wasn't figuring out what I needed to do for her; I knew what to do. Afterall I'd been her Mother now for over a year. The question was how I was going to do it. Feed her, bathe her, play with her, put her down for her nap, etc. I had to literally plan out how I was going to do those things when I didn't even have the energy to roll myself out of bed.  I had barely held my daughter the past couple of weeks.

Today, my fiancé was at work and I was on my own. Get it together, I told myself. You have a daughter that needs you. Though I was struggling, I fed her, bathed her, and took care of my baby. I wasn't tired, I was nauseous and very weak.

After giving my daughter a bath, I placed her in her swing, buckled her in and pulled the swing next to the couch where I could lay down and still be able to keep an eye on her. I had already thrown up a few times for the day and had nothing in my stomach. Being fully aware that even an empty stomach wouldn't stop me from throwing up, I placed a trash can next to the couch. I looked at the time and calculated my fiancé should be getting back in another hour or 2. Thank God, because I was feeling more and more miserable by the minute and was beginning to worry about being home alone with the baby.

I closed my eyes taking deep breaths trying to pass the time. A few minutes later, my daughter started crying. I reached over while still laying on the couch and tried to put her bottle in her mouth. But I couldn't reach.  I had to get up. All I remember was attempting to roll my body over to stand on my feet. The next thing I knew I was laying flat on the floor. My body was so weak that I couldn't move a muscle. Dazed, I could still hear my baby's cries getting louder and louder. "Get up, get up, get up", I told myself. But my body was not responding.

"Oh God, please don't let anything happen to her." I said out loud. What if she falls out of her swing? What if there's something seriously wrong with her? I was literally so weak that I couldn't even get up off the floor to pick up my own baby. Laying on the ground I started crying and can recall the tears barely being able to come out. What's happening to me?! I was petrified.

The next thing I recall is hearing my fiancé's voice. I opened my eyes and he was standing over me in the middle of the living room.

"What happened?" he asked me. He looked so nervous. I could still here our daughter crying. "Just pick her up, please. I can't move." I told him. He picked her up from the swing and she stopped crying almost immediately. She just needed to be held, I thought to myself while still in tears. I couldn't even hold my own baby.

As he helped me up off the floor and into bed, I felt completely helpless and inadequate. What kind of mother can't even take care of her own baby? What could have happened if he didn't come home when he did? I cried and cried and cried.

Lying in bed staring at the ceiling, I knew what I had to do. I had a daughter who needed her mother. When I decided to have her, I was also making it my life long obligation to be there for her, every day. But here I was leaving it all up to my fiancé because I didn't even have the strength to hold her. That wasn't fair. None of this was fair. But how do I explain sacrificing my unborn baby? I can't do that. It's not *his* fault! I did this. It's my body that's so messed up that I can't even perform the normal task of pregnancy. I can't do this to him! I cried and cried, again.

I laid there trying to think of an alternative. Maybe there was something else that can be done to help me have a healthy, normal pregnancy? Maybe I could hold on a little longer and this time it would go away and not last the entire pregnancy like it had before? Maybe there are other medications I could take? Maybe, maybe, maybe, kept running through my mind. But I knew in my gut nothing was going to get better.

Seeing this pregnancy through could mean not only putting myself at risk, but it would also put my unborn baby at risk as well. And what if I don't make it? A lot of people would lose, starting with my daughter. She would lose her Mother. I could possibly lose my life and that would mean my unborn baby wouldn't make it either. I know in life there are always choices, but this was one that I was not ever prepared to make.

The next day was Super Bowl Sunday. What would normally be a day filled with food, friends and fun, instead I literally spent the entire day in bed. Minus my visits to the bathroom sink. By 11pm I felt so physically ill that I decided to take myself to the local emergency room. Here we go again.

I asked my fiancé not to come with me. It was late, and I didn't want to wake our daughter, nor did I want her in the ER. Besides, I was already battling with an internal decision of what to do and I needed to go through the emotions alone. I had already discussed with him that I was considering terminating this pregnancy, and I just didn't want to pull him into what

I already felt was *my* mess. That might sound stupid and selfish, but it's how I felt. My body was the one going through it, so I would take on all the stress of this pregnancy myself.

A short cab ride later I was at the ER. "How far along are you?" asked the nurse. I replied that I'll be 10 weeks in a couple of days. While she was taking my vitals, the doctor came in and I explained my symptoms of constant nausea, vomiting, and feeling extremely weak. He started me on IV fluids while they ran blood and urine tests.

I laid alone in the room with a million thoughts running through my mind. I flashed back to the many hospital stays I had during my last pregnancy. I wondered how my fiancé was doing at home alone with our daughter. Hopefully she stayed asleep the entire night. I felt so guilty that I wasn't there with her. What seemed like only a few moments but was an hour later, the doctor returned and told me I was extremely dehydrated.

"I'm not surprised. I'm sure I am, doc." I replied recalling how many times I'd heard that during my last pregnancy. I haven't eaten, and I hadn't been drinking anything at all for days now. Being dehydrated didn't surprise me in the least. He also said I was running a fever which could mean I was also battling a stomach bug. My baby seemed to be doing well, despite everything my body was experiencing. Wanting to be certain, the doctor ordered a sonogram.

"Let's just make sure everything is OK in there. Just to be certain.", he said. Hesitantly, I agreed.

A sonogram? I didn't want to take another sonogram. For sure by now my baby had developed more than the last time I saw him on the monitor 3 weeks ago. I wasn't prepared to see him again. In my mind, I had already made the decision to terminate and seeing him would be devastating. It might even lead to me changing my mind and if I continued this pregnancy, I might not make it to the end. I can't look, I told myself. Just don't look.  Don't look.

Laying on the table, the technician began moving the probe across my belly. I turned my head to face the wall on the opposite direction of the sonogram screen. Don't look, just don't look, I kept telling myself.

"Ah, there he is!" the technician said eagerly.  "He's really moving around in there. Want to see?"

Ugh!  Why did he have to ask me that?! Of course, I wanted to look. I'm his mom. I know how amazing these moments can be. I know how incredible it was for your body to create life all on it's own and to see a tiny little person growing inside of you month by month. How could I not look? With tears already rolling down my eyes, I slowly turned my head to face my baby.

There *he* was. Alive. He was kicking, twisting and carrying on seemingly oblivious to what his mommy was going through. I swear I saw him sucking on his thumb. It reminded me of seeing my daughter during our doctor's visits. I cried even harder and fell in love with him immediately.

How dare I cry or even smile while looking at him? The guilt ran through my body like a heat flash.  I knew what I had already decided to do, and I felt I didn't have the right to love him. I didn't deserve his love. But I did. I couldn't help what I felt. My God, I loved my baby.

A few hours and 3 servings of IV fluids later, I was sent home with a prescription for Reglan, yet another anti-nausea medication. I was told to take Tylenol for the fever as needed, and Pepcid to provide some additional help combatting the nausea.

I got home at 4 in the morning. Obviously, after the night I had, there was no way I could make it to work. While being home alone, I vowed I would give this new medication a shot at making me feel better. Then I would make my final decision on whether to terminate. I prayed for it to work. I couldn't stand the thought of terminating, but I couldn't envision myself surviving this pregnancy either.

I called my mom that afternoon. I had been afraid to talk to her because although I would tell her I was OK, she would always see right through me. It's a mom thing, I guess. I couldn't lie to her even when I tried. She had only recently accepted the fact that I was going to take a gamble at yet another difficult pregnancy and although she never said it, I knew it was breaking her heart.

My mom always wanted me to have children so that she can spoil them rotten. But my last pregnancy had scared her so much that she just didn't want to see me go through that again. I wasn't prepared for the reaction she was going to give me on the phone that day when I shared with her that I was thinking of terminating. If anyone knows my mom, you'd know that she was deep in her Catholic beliefs and terminations are just never an option. Her response to me when I shared my thoughts, were shocking.

"Mom, I don't think I can do this. My body just doesn't respond well to pregnancy and this time it's even worse than before. I feel like I'm not going to make it."

I waited for her to respond. Her silence on the other

end seemed so loud. I guess she didn't make it off the phone quickly enough this time because she began crying hysterically. "I'm sorry, Mom. I'm so sorry." I said, thinking she was crying at my heinous thoughts to terminate.

But instead, she replied through her cries "Please, just do it. If you're going to do it, just do it now while it's still early. I don't want to lose you. I have a feeling you're going to *die* if you continue this pregnancy."

I sat on the phone in shock. This was not what I expected to hear. I think I was hoping she'd talk me out of it so that I would have the courage to keep going. But hearing my Mother sobbing on the phone pierced my heart like a hot knife. Her cries sounded like she was already grieving my death. If even my Mother, the most God-fearing woman I knew was supporting me with this decision, I knew I was doing worse than I thought.

I pictured my fiancé having to raise our daughter on his own. I pictured him mourning my loss and the loss of our unborn baby. I pictured my mother falling so deep into a state of depression after losing me, that she wouldn't live much longer herself. Then my daughter, Isabelle. I sat there and pictured her life without me. Without her Mother. The woman who gave her life simultaneously promising to be there for her until the end of her own life. Now I was putting myself in the position where she may have to grow up only knowing her Mother through pictures and stories. I knew what I had to do, but doing it wasn't going to be easy.

The next day, I called and made an appointment to terminate. The night before going in, I didn't sleep a wink. I stared into the darkness sinking deeper and deeper into a state of depression. I was a Mother and in hours I was going to allow someone to kill my baby. Let's just call a spade a spade, right? I had to accept and take responsibility for my decisions. Still sick and feeling like I was losing my breath with every attempt I took of inhaling, I got out of bed and crawled into the bathroom. After throwing up I sat in the dark on the cold bathroom floor and sobbed like a child.

"I'm sorry, baby. Mommy is so very sorry. I'm sorry I wasn't good enough. I'm sorry that I have to do this. I love you. Please know that Mommy loves you and none of this was your fault. I'm sorry Mommy's body isn't strong enough to keep you safe. I'm sorry. I'm so sorry." I must have repeated that a million times that night.

I cried on the floor for hours. The tears wouldn't let up. I was so disappointed in myself, in my body. How can I not be woman enough to handle this? I felt as though I was sacrificing the life of one child for another. What type of mother makes a decision like that? A mother who wanted to survive for her child, I guess. The child she had already made the promise to be there for. It wasn't fair. Life at that moment just didn't make any sense.

Still laying on the floor, it dawned on me that I never had the chance to give me unborn baby a name. It was still too early to know what I was having, but in my heart, I always felt like it was a boy. My sweet thumb-sucking little boy. You will not be nameless in heaven, I thought to myself.

Without having to think too hard, I knew what his name would be. Tristan. I shared the same name as my mother, Yseult, which her father had named her from an old romantic tale of Tristan and Yseult, spelled Isolde in Irish. The story goes that Tristan and Yseult were so in love with each other, but Yseult was already promised to another. There are several versions of this tale of love and tragedy, but there was one that always stood out for me. The 2 were so in love and saddened by never being able to be together, that Tristan eventually dies from grief and Yseult cried over his body, grieving his loss forever. The story was fitting, and so was the name. With one hand on my belly, I stood up and whispered in the dark, "Your name is Tristan, my baby."

The morning came quickly. The worst snow storm of the season had started overnight. My fiancé was up taking care of our daughter as I got myself ready for my appointment. We had already spoken the night before and I explained why I didn't want him there with me. It was something I felt I needed to endure alone. Although it was our baby, it was *my* baby. I needed to take this on alone.

Soon, I was headed to the clinic in a cab. It felt like we were the only ones on the road. The snow was falling so heavily that my cabdriver could barely see past the hood of his own car. There was no one else on the road. Only us. There were so many moments when I felt like asking him to please turn around. But every time I thought of saying something, my daughter's face would appear in my mind. Remember why you're doing this, I would remind myself. Then quietly I would sit back, close my eyes and pray.

When I finally arrived, I was surprised to walk into a small room with at least 8 other women already waiting. I guess I wasn't the only one crazy enough to battle a storm today. I was seen by a few different staff members before finally going in for what I came there for. I entered a room with a female technician ready to perform a final sonogram.

"Hello, how are you?" she asked me nicely. Do you really want to know? I wanted to respond. "I'm OK", I replied instead. I don't know how, but we managed to get on the topic of morning sickness. I told her how miserable my pregnancy has been with persistent nausea and vomiting.

"You should try eating raw ginger. My sister was the same way and that helped her a lot." she said. Was this lady freaking kidding me?! Was she unaware of where she worked? What I was there to do? The amount of strength I had to muster up to come in and do all alone just to hear her now giving me advice on what I could do to make my nausea better?! Doesn't she know I've tried everything under the sun including taking a ton of potentially dangerous medications that could harm my baby, just so that I could try to see this pregnancy through to the end? Was she seriously giving me advice right now? Screaming all of these thoughts inside my head I calmly replied "I've tried that too. Nothing works for me." At least she wasn't dumb enough to show me the sonogram screen.

Moments later I was being escorted into another room. Now dressed in a hospital gown, I had flashbacks of having my daughter. But obviously, this experience wasn't going to be the same. I remember the nurse that day. I remembered that she couldn't pronounce my name. So instead of trying she just yelled out "next" like we **were** waiting to place a food order. I was so afraid. Not for me, but for my baby. I had done a fine job at traumatizing myself by watching way too many videos on the termination process, so I was way to familiar with what happens next. I didn't want him to feel any pain.

The room was cold, but my nerves were what was causing me to tremble uncontrollably. The nurse asked me to lay on the table face up and to slide my body all the way down to the end. Like the position you lay in while being examined by your Gynecologist. Just then a doctor walked in. I can't remember his face at all, only that there was a certain coldness about him.

"Do you have any questions?" he calmly asked me while standing 2 feet away looking down at his notepad. He never made eye contact with me.

"No" I replied, my voice cracking. I reached into my bag of belongings that were sitting on top of the table next to me and grabbed my rosary. I wrapped it around my left hand and placed my right hand on my belly as the nurse began administering the anesthesia, the tears began to fall down my cheeks. "I'm so sorry" I whispered, as my eyes closed.

It felt like I had just closed my eyes for a moment but about 20 minutes had gone already by. I woke up in another room surrounded by several other women laying or sitting up in their hospital gowns. A few of them were snacking on chips and drinking juice or water. I looked down at my left hand and realized my rosary had broken in half. How did that happen, I asked myself? Why would anyone do that? Immediately, the guilt hit me. I felt it was a sign that I had done something so wrong and there was no coming back from it. You know what felt even crazier than that? My nausea, it was completely gone. I felt, nothing. I felt empty. It hit me that my baby was gone.

I cried for an hour in that recover room. I was the only one crying. Embarrassed, I tried several times to use the sheet that was covering me with the intentions of keeping me warm to instead hide my face with it.

But every time a nurse would walk by and ask me to lower it. I felt so ashamed. They had me wait a couple of hours before letting me go. I was prescribed Ibuprofen 800 mg for the pain. I never took a single dose. I felt I deserved the pain, so I decided I would just suffer my way through it.

Returning home that afternoon, I didn't really say much. My fiancé gave me a long hug when I walked in and asked me if I was OK. I nodded, bent down to kiss my daughter on the forehead who was quietly napping in her crib and went straight to bed.

I slept for hours. I woke up starving and felt guilty for wanting food. I hadn't eaten much of anything in days and whatever I ate came right back out. So now that I wasn't nauseous anymore, my body needed food to recover. Still feeling guilty about it, I ate some of the pasta my fiancé had ordered for me.

The next day without missing a beat, I went back to work. Shocked to see me getting ready in the morning, my fiancé asked me "Are you sure you don't want to take another day off?" He knew I needed time to heal physically and emotionally I was a wreck.

"No, I'm going to work" I told him. "I just killed my baby so that I could be here and feel better. I don't deserve anymore days off. I won't let his sacrifice go in vein."

### ***HYPEREMESIS GRAVIDARUM***

**Definition:** severe, excessive form of morning **sickness** (nausea, vomiting) associated with **weight loss & imbalance of electrolytes in the blood.** Develops during 1st or 2nd trimester (persists >16 weeks gestation). Hyperemesis = excessive vomiting.

**Pathophysiology:** increased sensitivity in the

vomiting center of the brain to the increasing hormones of pregnancy (e.g., beta-hCG). The 4 chemicals in our brain that directly cause nausea and/or vomiting are serotonin, histamine, acetylcholine and dopamine so medications work by blocking these chemicals that trigger nausea and/or vomiting.

**Who's At Risk:** previous hyperemesis in past pregnancy, multiple gestations, molar pregnancy (a type of abnormal pregnancy), migraine suffers.

**Clinical Manifestations:** nausea and or vomiting. **Hyperemesis gravidarum is associated with more severe symptoms, weight loss** of 5% of pre-pregnant weight, acidosis (buildup of acid in the blood from starvation).

**When To Call Your Doctor:** if you develop weight loss, vomiting is excessive, you develop weakness or muscle cramps, the symptoms are worsening or persisting.

**Management:** All management options should be discussed with your primary care giver. Options include but are not limited to:

**Lifestyle modifications:** **ginger**, high protein foods, small and frequent meals, avoiding trigger goods (e.g., spicy or fatty foods), increasing fluid intake. Women can keep a diarrhea of triggers and foods that may provoke nausea and vomiting.

• **Pyridoxine (vitamin B6) with or without Doxylamine** is often **first-line medical management.**

• If no relief, antihistamines can be used (e.g., Dimenhydrinate, Meclizine or Diphenhydramine).

• 3rd line: dopamine-blocking agents (e.g., Metoclopramide or Promethazine). Ondansetron (serotonin blockers).

• If decreased volume occurs, intravenous fluids and electrolyte replacement. May need Dimenhydrinate, Meclizine, Diphenhydramine. Ondansetron if severe vomiting.

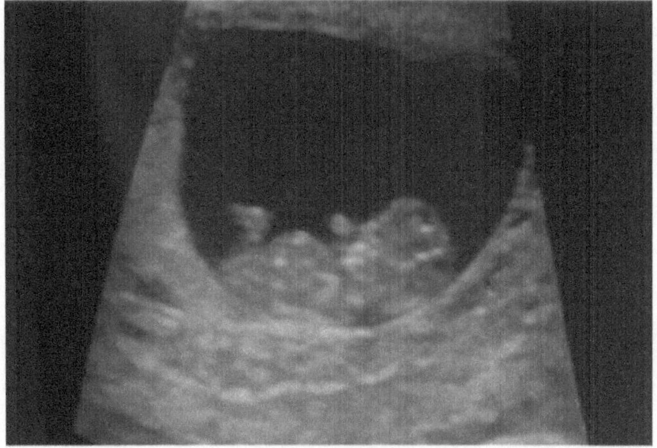

**Tristan David Rowan**

# *15*

# HEALING

A month later I followed up with my GYN. Making the call to his office for an appointment after the termination was so difficult. Everyone there knew me well, so when I called, they immediately asked me how I was feeling and how the baby was doing. Having to tell them I had terminated my pregnancy was rough, but they weren't the least bit surprised. I guess they saw what I was going through and how rough pregnancy was for me.

I sat with my doctor and told him all about my experience. I asked to start on birth control again immediately. I used to take birth control religiously many years ago but had decided to give my body a break for a while. I suffered from chronic migraines and the hormones from the birth control made them worse.

As horrible as those migraines were, nothing was worse than what my body endured with pregnancy and I promised myself never to go through that again.

"Can you please tie my tubes now?" I asked him. "You're still young and that requires major surgery", he replied.

Considering I've had abdominal surgery several times before, the risks from performing that procedure were just too high. So, I decided I'd have to be on birth control until menopause.

I had several months of healing ahead of me. Not just my body, but I also had a lot of mental and emotional healing I needed to do. After the termination, I fell into another deep state of depression. It was so hard sometimes to snap myself out of it. I had to just keep reminding myself why I decided to do what I did, and I spent every moment I could with my daughter. Not only giving her back the time we had missed together but devoting myself to being even more present in her life. Friends who knew what I had gone through would tell me to just look at her pretty little face whenever I felt like I couldn't go on, and that helped me a lot.

Physically, my body had gone through so much and I needed to give myself the time it needed to heal. Mentally, I found it helpful jotting down my feelings as I was going through my healing process. When I felt like crying, I cried. When I felt like smiling, I did. Eventually, I stopped allowing the guilt of what I did run my life. Again, I refused to let *him* losing his life be in vein. I allowed myself to learn from both experiences and to grow from them.

My emotions would prove to be the hardest hurdle to overcome. I wondered, how can I help myself heal? I couldn't control what I was feeling, nor could I stop myself from having emotions. So, I had to figure out a way help myself heal emotionally.

I wondered if there was anyone out there who had gone through what I went through or something similar. I began to think how alone I felt with both pregnancies. All I wanted was something, or someone to tell me that I wasn't alone in this struggle called pregnancy. How could I help someone else going through a rough pregnancy? How can I help them not feel so alone? Then one morning it hit me… I'm going to share my story with the world.

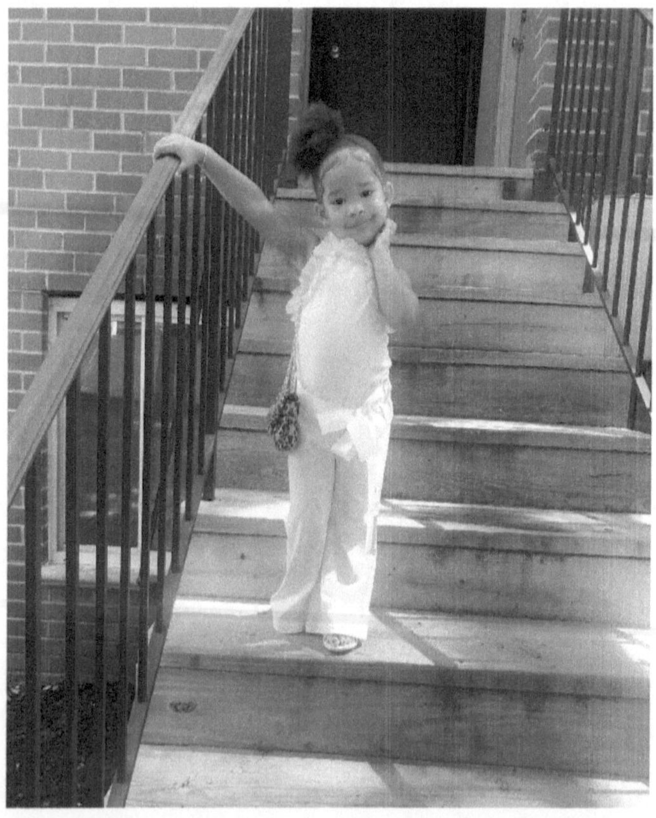

**Isabelle Casey Rowan at 3 years old.**

**Disclaimer: The medical information provided in this book is not intended to be nor should it replace or determine a medical diagnosis.  It is important that you consult with your physician to determine the best course of action for your individual pregnancy.**